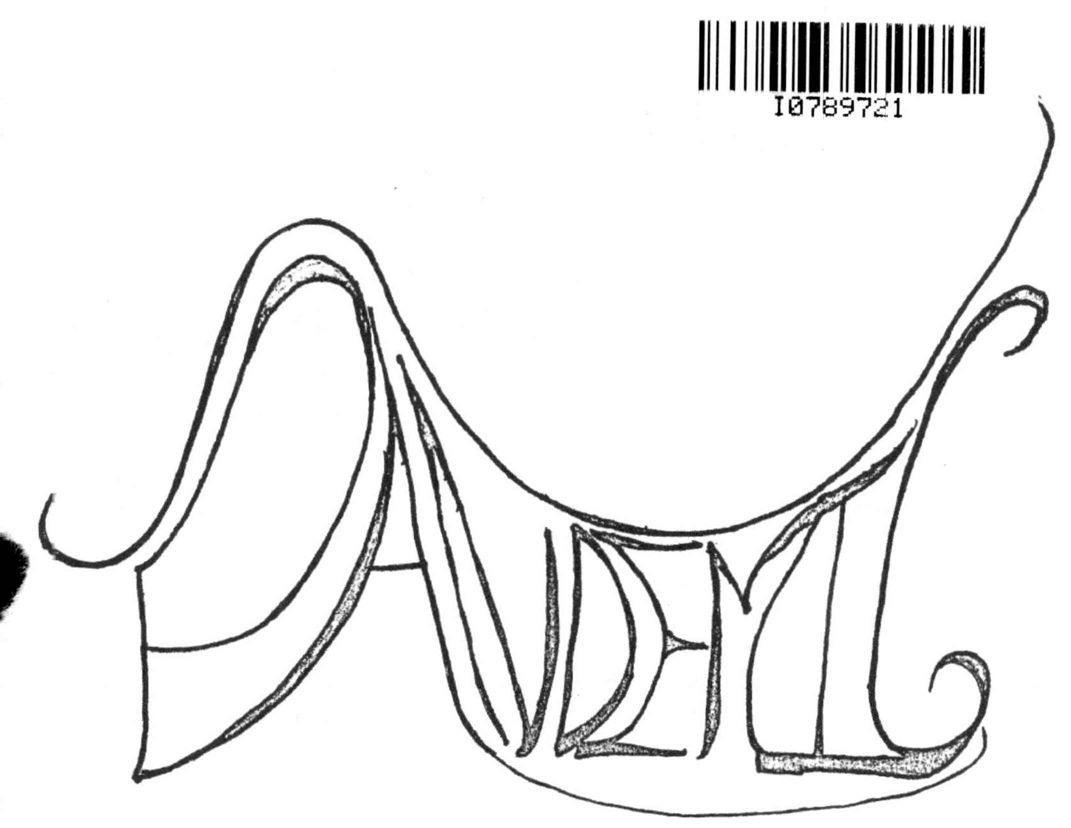

PANDEMIC MANIFESTO

1ST EDITION

COVID-19 BASIC TRAINING FROM THE FRONTLINES

FACE THE NEXT PANDEMIC FROM A POSITION OF POWER

BY

DR. FARAH FOURCAND, MD

DEDICATIONS

The Legendary Five

Extubation Day April 17, 2020 will live on forever.

.-.. --- ...- .

The COVID-19 Brain Team

Your anti-inflammatory response to the cytokine storm of the century

was superhero-worthy.

.-. . ... .--. . -.-. -

Kathryn & Kraig

#melatonin

..-. .-. .. . -. -.. ... .--.

TABLE OF CONTENTS

PREFACE. THE SILVER LINING — 1

OPENING REMARKS. TREAD CONFIDENTLY WITH YOUR WISDOM STICK — 5

I. KNOW THE ENEMY. POWER IN NUMBERS & STRENGTH IN DIVERSITY — 8

II. TO FLATTEN THE CURVE. EPIDEMIC CURVES, MITIGATION & PPE — 11

III. GATEKEEPER DEFENSE. ANTIBODIES, ACE, REINFECTION & BAD TESTS — 22

IV. THERE WILL BE BLOOD. BLOOD TYPE, CLOTS, SPIKE & ECMO — 27

V. I AM THE STORM. CYTOKINE STORMING & COVID-19 BIOMARKERS — 32

VI. WAR PROPAGANDA. THE MISEDUCATION OF QT & HYDROXYCHLOROQUINE — 36

VII. DECLASSIFIED INFORMATION. VACCINES & HOW CLINICAL TRIALS WORK — 40

VIII. DRUG ARSENAL. PLASMA, TOCILIZUMAB, REMDESIVIR & CO. — 46

IX. ALCHEMY NOW. MELATONIN, VITAMIN D & ZINC + C — 50

X. THE GREAT DICTATOR. VENTILATORS, PRONING, ARDS, HPV & HAPE!#%&$? — 54

XI. ORGAN STRIKE. KIDNEY PUNCH, GUTS & THE MEDULLA OBLONGATA — 60

XII. CASUALTIES OF WAR. TESTOSTERONE, YOUTH, KAWASAKI & COVID TOES — 66

XIII. PSYCHOLOGICAL WARFARE. SURVIVAL OF THE WELL-ADJUSTED — 71

CLOSING REMARKS. BUILD A VAST MEMORY PALACE — 75

BIBLIOGRAPHY — 77

ACKNOWLEDGEMENTS — 96

ABOUT THE AUTHOR — 97

PREFACE

THE SILVER LINING

DEFINITIONS

Intubation (Noun): Semi-reversible process of inserting a breathing tube attached to a ventilator into the airway of a person unable to protect it. *Verb: To intubate.*

Extubation (Noun): The glorious and gross process of removing a breathing tube attached to a ventilator from a person's airway after scrupulous evaluation. *Verb: To extubate.*

Pulse oximeter or 'ox' (Noun): A clothespin-like sensor placed on part of the body far away from the heart, typically a finger or nostril, which is a good estimate of the body's oxygen level. *Abbreviation: SpO2.*

Arterial blood gas or 'ABG' (Noun): Artery blood test that measures pH, carbon dioxide, oxygen, and bicarbonate levels to determine if an abnormality in the acid-base balance of the lungs and body exists. *Readout: $pH/pCO_2/PaO_2/HCO_3/SpO_2$.*

Centrifugation (Noun): A spinning technique used to separate blood into red blood cells and plasma at speeds of up to 20,000 RPM. *Verb: To centrifuge.*

It was 0600 on a Friday in the old Neuro ICU as I walked into a modern-day warzone: the COVID-19 ICU. Of the 300+ COVID-19 patients occupying our 499-bed hospital, nearly 100 were on the ventilator. Twenty of the sickest COVID-19 patients, many of whom had been on the ventilator for weeks, were housed in the old Neuro ICU I still called home. Needless to say, that as neurocritical care, neurointerventional surgery, and neurosurgery doctors now redeployed as COVID-19 frontliners, the learning curve was steep. Nevertheless, as part of the COVID-19 'Brain Team,' I volunteered to step up and out of my comfort zone to fight alongside fellow frontline healthcare workers.

To put things in perspective, by most projections less than 1% of people with COVID-19 are hospitalized. Approximately 10% of people sick enough to be hospitalized need to be intubated and placed on the ventilator, and up to 90% of ventilator-dependent patients die[a]. Thousands of COVID-19 patients have been discharged from hospitals but were rarely, if ever, critically ill and ventilator-dependent. But, herein lies the silver lining. On a day like any other, at the peak of the COVID-19 pandemic in an epicenter microcosm plagued by the same hurdles and hardships as anywhere else, a rare feat was accomplished. Five of 20, or 25%, of patients in the old Neuro ICU were extubated in one day. This is my story.

0545: I woke up late, and for a few precious seconds I forgot I was in a quarantine hotel bed. I *finally* had a good night's sleep. Shortness of breath following a COVID-19 exposure and breach of PPE that plagued me the last few nights had finally resolved. I put on my uniform, found a makeshift pulse ox crafted for me by Dr. M and Jacqueline, and smiled. On the drive, I reminisced about the small milestones I missed since being away from my family. After my temperature was checked at the ER entrance, I gathered PPE from Special Procedures and, with 5 minutes to spare, I scavenged the hospital for espresso, half-and-half, and sugar to customize my morning coffee. I managed to balance my oversized COVID-19 clinical trial folder, liquid breakfast, and protective gear while running up the stairs and smizing through my facemask at passersby, all of whom were unrecognizable in full PPE camo. And then, like clockwork "Rapid Response Team needed STAT, Intubation Team needed STAT, and Code Blue Team needed STAT" blared overhead on repeat loop. I took a deep breath, donned my N-95, surgeon's cap, face shield, and badged into the COVID-19 ICU.

0615: As I tactically walked into a minefield, I bore witness to the fresh wounds inflicted in the night. In the aftermath of two young patients unexpectedly losing their battle against COVID-19, I overheard a few nurses to my left entertaining the idea of quitting nursing. To my right, Cleopatra, a well-respected teaching nurse, tearfully led a prayer group. Straight ahead, a crew of redeployed army nurses and a pair of correctional officers safeguarding intubated COVID-19 inmates vented about the audacity of people broadcasting the woes and boredom of quarantine. My senior co-fellow and I walked around the unit for checkout rounds, and I noticed that even his typically grounded, levelheaded demeanor was shaken.

0630: I gowned up and entered the room of the first extubation candidate. I changed his ventilator settings to challenge him to breathe on his own, temporarily stopped his tube feeds to prevent aspiration, and lowered his sedation to gauge his level of alertness and give a heartfelt "you can do it" game day pep talk. I proceeded to de-gown, re-gown, and repeat. For the 5 out of 7 who passed the test, an ABG and chest x-ray were ordered to give my pie-in-the-sky optimism real-world perspective.

0800: In the meantime, Dr. K and I tended to the needs of the 15 other patients who would hopefully have their day in the metaphorical sun too. "Patient A has a pulmonary embolism and needs TPA and a heparin drip, Patient B is no longer a candidate for remdesivir because of worsening kidney function, Patient C's chest tubes have an air leak, Patient X needs central and arterial lines, Patient Y has a pH of 6.66, fever of 109°F, and needs a second vasopressor…god help us, and so on" I remember nonchalantly reading back while, in reality, my mind was running a mile a minute. Amidst the pandemonium, two STAT intubations from earlier were wheeled in to fill the two empty beds of our dearly and prematurely departed. While piecemealing together histories of a Times Square COVID-19 exposure and yet another mysterious pre-COVID-19 illness, I returned messages from team members not physically on service, who nevertheless remained a constant presence. Dr. S, pre-COVID-19 neurosurgeon and newly appointed ventilator Jedi, followed up to ensure a patient was weaned off APRV ventilator mode and proned. Dr. Z, who took the lead in a COVID-19 convalescent plasma study, reassured us he made headway in urgently getting plasma to our patients. He was committed to doing so sooner than later in an effort to beat the disease rather than chase it because, in his own words, "it sucks to play Monday morning quarterback."

1000: "Every patient gets Decadron 10mg IV, Ritalin 10mg OG, Robinul 2mg IV, a Scopolamine patch, BIPAP at 14 over 6, and nebulizer treatments ready as backup" Dr. K announced. He recapitulated the importance of double dotting I's and triple crossing T's by broadening antibiotics, correcting blood sugars, normalizing blood pressures, balancing electrolytes, optimizing fluid statuses, et cetera to ensure that this series of small miracles went off without a hitch. In a toxically grim climate amongst those overwhelmed with work and underwhelmed with outcomes, healthcare worker morale was depending on it.

1159: As the first patient was extubated, his nurse Fernanda, Dr. K, and myself surrounded his bed in an almost ritualistic configuration. The patient, a middle-aged man who overcame COVID-19-related kidney failure, breathed room air for the first time in weeks and half-smiled as we ceremoniously applauded him. Out of the corner of my eye, I caught curious glances from outside the negative pressure room. We then made our way back to the workstation to regroup, put out fires, and do damage control. Dr. I, Gina, and Anna stopped by to let us know they placed dialysis catheters in two of our COVID-19 patients with acute kidney failure before rushing to a neurosurgical emergency.

1230: With an increasing number of skeptical followers, Dr. K and I continued to make our extubation rounds. The second patient cared for by Renee woke up enough to be extubated after hearing his daughter on the phone. We then headed to the infamous 'back desk.' A young man with a telenovela-worthy backstory was extubated third. An elderly man we took a chance on because he always looked better in person than on electronic paper was extubated fourth. Another elderly man who survived septic shock and blood clots was extubated fifth after being teed up the entire day by his no-nonsense nurse Lauren. I now recall how serendipitous it was that Mike, our head respiratory therapist, unintentionally pushed up our ventilator 'weaning timeline' and wished he were there to see how the stars had aligned on this special day. In the surreal moments that followed, we called loved ones, none of whom were allowed to visit. The emotions on the other end of the line were palpable, and the positivity in the air was contagious.

1700: After five extubations and well past our shift, Dr. K and I headed back to the Neuroscience Institute to work on our COVID-19 clinical trial. We performed COVID-19 testing on the study's first subject, my brave senior co-fellow, who volunteered to be the guinea pig for us to practice the performance art of nasal swabbing and plasma centrifugation before going live. On our way back to the COVID-19 ICU we realized that, akin to the best game of telephone ever, word of the extubations spread like wildfire. Within hours, every doctor, nurse, and staff member had caught wind of the small cohort of hope in the old Neuro ICU.

1900: I headed to the ICU break room to give social distancing-approved air hugs to nurses moved by the day's events and to have my first meal in 24 hours. I closed my eyes and imagined the leftover donated pizza from lunch was hot, fresh chicaronnes and pastelitos (yes, I'm a Miami girl). On my way out, I greeted Peter, our superhuman clinical pharmacist, who undoubtedly burned the midnight oil coordinating study drug logistics. I interrupted his workflow to remind him of the good news and confirmed my inkling that only *some* but not all of the extubated patients had actually received a special, coveted study drug. In the locker room, I changed out of my dirty scrubs, stared into the mirror, and owned my PPE 'acne-esque' battle scars. I drove back to the quarantine hotel anticipating the nostalgia I would always have for this day.

2200: I remembered to FaceTime my family to ask about their day but did not have the mental energy or heart to talk candidly about mine. I went on Facebook to reply to a friend's COVID-19-related question from two weeks earlier (I know, facepalm) and saw that Tina, a Neuro ICU nurse redeployed to one of the dozen or so units converted to a COVID-19 ICU, posted "for the first time I cried tears of joy instead of tears of sadness on my drive home after hearing the good news." Suddenly, I was reinvigorated. I reheated stale popcorn and started brainstorming about a COVID-19 'Crash Course.' About one sentence in, I realized I was all smoke and no fire. And so, right before passing out, I proceeded to text Dr. Z to find out if anyone was re-intubated. No one was. Take that, COVID-19. Lights out.

REFERENCE

[a] Safiya Richardson, Jamie S. Hirsch, Mangala Narasimhan, James M. Crawford, Thomas McGinn, Karina W. Davidson. Presenting Characteristics, Comorbidities, and Outcomes Among 5700 Patients Hospitalized With COVID-19 in the New York City Area. *JAMA*, 2020; 323(20): 2052-2059. doi:10.1001/jama.2020.6775.

OPENING REMARKS
TREAD CONFIDENTLY WITH YOUR WISDOM STICK

Without training, they lacked knowledge.
Without knowledge, they lacked confidence.
Without confidence, they lacked victory.

—Julius Caesar
Historian, Statesman, General & Mastermind Behind the Rise of the Roman Empire

The purpose of this manifesto is to teach you *how to fish* for accurate and reliable information today, tomorrow, and beyond. In a sea of misinformation, it is nearly impossible to find no-nonsense, science-driven, evidence-based information you need to walk humbly in your knowledge and carry a big stick of your wisdom. Case in point: COVID-19.

From hearsay on its origins, mental and physical unpreparedness for its impact, and socioeconomic and philosophical quagmires in its aftermath, a most fundamental principle has been lost. What is the Achilles heel of the pathogen archetype, whether we are facing the Bubonic Plague, Spanish Flu, or COVID-19? Answering this question will provide you with a roadmap to navigate almost any medical mystery, empower you with knowledge to face the next pandemic with objective eyes, enhance your general understanding of medicine, and instill in you the confidence to not let uncertainty and change be purveyors of fear and intimidation. The quest for this answer motivated me to not just survive but thrive during these challenging times, and I want to help you do the same. But first, a fair warning on what is fair game:

Out of respect and transparency for the educated citizens who by way of finding this text have already added a long list of scientific and medical terms to their fund of knowledge, this manifesto is written to be explanatory _and_ challenging. And so, please do the following:
   ◊   Read in order from cover to cover.
   ◊   Read slowly and deliberately.
   ◊   Be patient. Trust me; I understand your frustrations…

Pre-COVID-19, I was the only woman in my stroke, neurocritical care, and neurointerventional surgery program and, of course, I had my work cut out for me. After beating the odds to get into college, medical school, residency, and a competitive research program at the NIH to be where I was when COVID-19 hit, a pandemic derailing my training and my life blindsided me to say the least. And yet, nothing ever motivated me more than this experience to step up and out of my comfort zone, surpass a steep learning curve, and think for myself in the absence of evidence and evidence of urgency. As you probably gathered from my *Silver Lining* story, I am honored to have been part of the COVID-19 Brain Team and never felt more like a doctor. This once-in-a-lifetime experience motivated me to start COVID-19 'Crash Course,' usually recorded raw and unedited from my iPhone around 0300 in the COVID-19 ICU or my quarantine hotel room. Appreciation from its very small following served as the impetus for this manifesto. Here, we take a deeper dive into a full gamut of matters relevant to any viral outbreak, epidemic, or pandemic we may encounter in our lifetimes.

Information is fluid, especially in these dynamic times. That being said, the importance of evidence-based medicine *is* emphasized throughout this text. However, frontline experience comes close to trumping evidence in the current pandemic because of logistical barriers in clinical trial design and the adulteration of science by political underpinnings. Therefore, many references in this manifesto refer to well-conceptualized studies that may not necessarily be randomized controlled trials or meta-analyses. Even the current COVID-19 'clinical guidelines' and 'critical appraisals' of the literature are admittedly premature and change day-to-day. And so, let principles and methodology not minutia imprint upon you by not letting the devil in the details obscure your view of the forest beyond the trees.

And remember, wars were fought long before humankind took foothold and patented the trademark. Here, we are fighting a war against a microscopic entity that has inflicted very real wounds on humankind at large by means of exposing our own fears, limitations, and vulnerabilities. In essence, COVID-19 is winning a war it was never equipped to fight in the first place. And so, read every word herein written, and then, please think for yourself.

Godspeed, and stay informed.

The Pyramid of Evidence. As you search for answers from today onward and long after you read this manifesto, do so using the strategic approach: evidence-based medicine. In the heat of the moment and reality of the times, the highest level of evidence is sometimes unavailable and unrealistic as is the case in COVID-19. But, by using sound judgement and your proverbial wisdom stick, you will find a happy medium of truth.

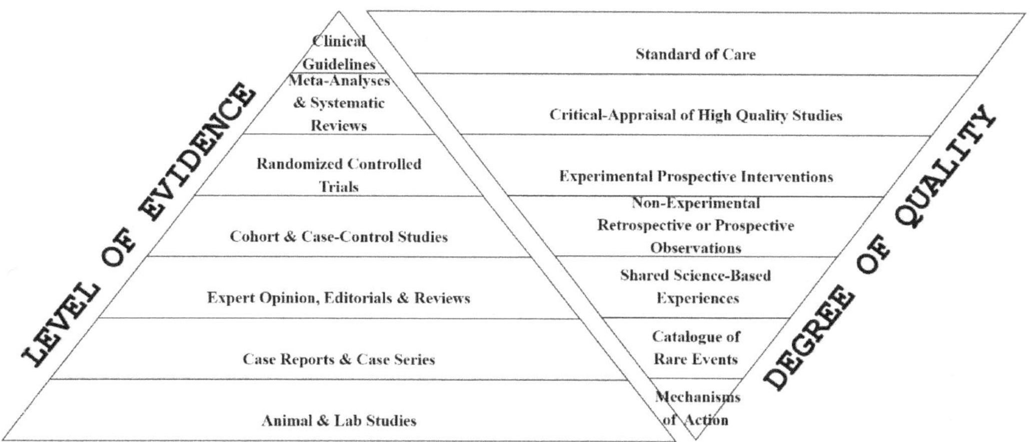

<u>Warning</u>: With rare exceptions, information presented via hot-off-the-press release and non-expert/pseudoscience opinion is neither evidence-based science nor real medicine.

I. Know The (microscopic) Enemy

Power In Numbers & Strength In Diversity

It is said that if you know the enemy and know yourself, you need not fear the result of a hundred battles. If you know yourself but not the enemy, for every victory gained you will also suffer a defeat. If you know neither the enemy nor yourself, you will succumb in every battle.

—The Art of War by Sun Tzu
  Chinese General, Military Strategist & Philosopher

Each of us is a singular representative of the human species. Likewise, each bacterium and virus in the human body and in nature is a discrete entity, representative of its species. In the human body, it is thought that bacterial cells outnumber human cells 10 to 1, or 100 trillion to 10 trillion. Although recent studies suggest less skewed differences[1], this does not take into account other microbes and the even *more* microscopic viruses housed in the human body. And so, in order to gain perspective and visualize the enemy, we will keep things simple.

These trillions (or quadrillions) of microbes are akin to an army of individual organisms within one human body. The human 'microbiome' is a community of bacteria, fungi, viruses, bacteriophages (viruses that infection bacteria), and archaea (organisms that blur the microbe line and live in extreme environments) in the body. The human body is 100,000 times larger than a human cell with the exception of a human egg cell that is wider than a human hair and the 3-feet-long sciatic nerves that course down from spine to feet. The human body is 1 million times larger than a bacterial cell, and a bacterial cell is 10 times smaller than a human cell. And, if you can imagine, the human body is 10 million times larger than a virus, and a virus is 100 times smaller than a human cell. This begs the question as to why the uber-microscopic world has such a foothold in ours. Well, there is power in numbers.

As stated above, microbes outnumber human cells at least 10 to 1. As such, microbes heavily influence the human condition, from immune defense to neural network communication. The influence of viruses in particular is even more elusive. While bacteria and most other microbes are quarantined to their own quarters in the human body, viruses infiltrate human cells because they are unable to live outside of their host. After a virus invades, if it does not conquer, it hides in plain sight and lies in wait until its host is vulnerable. At that time, it colludes with its viral brethren and takes formation into a 'Trojan Horse' attacking from the inside out.

Just as not all bacteria are pathogenic, or 'pathological,' not all viruses are virulent, or 'violent' in nature. There are an estimated 1,000 bacterial species in the human body with 2,000 genes per species, or a composite of 2 million genes. This is 100 times the number of human genes estimated to be 20,000. The diversity of viruses in the human body is unknown, but just as they outrank bacteria in number, they presumably outnumber in diversity of species. From the era of the Human Genome[2] and Microbiome[3] Projects, the Global Virome Project[4] has recently emerged in humankind's attempt to gain the upper hand on the microscopic battlefield. Now, one may ask how humans accomplish such great feats, some of which are literally otherworldly, but cannot defeat a rogue micro-villain.

Think again of the enemy: 10 million times smaller than the human body and 100 times smaller than a human cell. Appreciate the technology needed to even fathom observation of the enemy. As a refresher, atoms (basic units of matter) are 1,000 times smaller than a virus. The atom's constituents (protons, neutrons, and electrons) are 100,000 times smaller than their parent atom. This is the same size ratio as the human body to human cell: 100,000 to 1. It follows that, if you throw yourself into the limbo of inception, the microscope needed to examine a human cell needs its own microscope to examine a virus, ergo the electron microscope. And as you know, observation rests just at the surface of knowing the enemy.

A virus is only 10 to 50 times larger than a strand of DNA, the carrier of all genetic information. As such, viruses are defined by whether they are made of DNA or RNA. RNA is the mirror image of DNA that sends messages and signals to DNA outside of the cell core, or nucleus. Coronaviruses are a family of RNA viruses that resemble a *corona*, or crown, under an electron microscope. Their hosts are mammals and birds, and seven types of coronaviruses are known to infect humans. Two viruses cause the common cold, one virus causes community-acquired pneumonia, and one virus causes bronchitis.

The other three coronaviruses are rare and sometimes fatal. The virus MERS-CoV causes the disease Middle East respiratory syndrome, or MERS. The virus SARS-CoV causes the disease severe acute respiratory syndrome, or SARS. And, last but certainly not least, SARS-CoV-2 causes the disease CoronaVirus Disease 2019, or COVID-19. The subtle point here is that a virus and disease are not synonymous. An enemy virus such as SARS-CoV-2 infects a host and, depending on a *host* of host defenses, causes or does not cause a disease such as COVID-19. Throughout this manifesto, previous knowledge of MERS and SARS, as well as several other viruses, will be used to predict mechanisms of action and outcomes in COVID-19. As members of the same family, SARS-CoV-2 shares approximately 79% of its genes with SARS-CoV and 52% of its genes with MERS-CoV[5]. Many of the genetic differences in SARS-CoV-2 compared to its viral kin are related to its enhanced *virulent* properties.

I digress. Indeed, the enemy is enormously small. But, as we now know, the most vulnerable amongst us are vastly outnumbered and under-diversified. Now, we will turn our focus from introspective examination of the enemy's microenvironment to root-cause analyses of the human host defense starting with our efforts in macroscopic mitigation: flattening the curve.

Microscopic Inception. A visual representation of relative sizes and diversity of the microscopic world within the human body. From outer circle to inner circle: human cell, bacterial cell, virus, DNA and RNA, atoms, and subatomic matter.

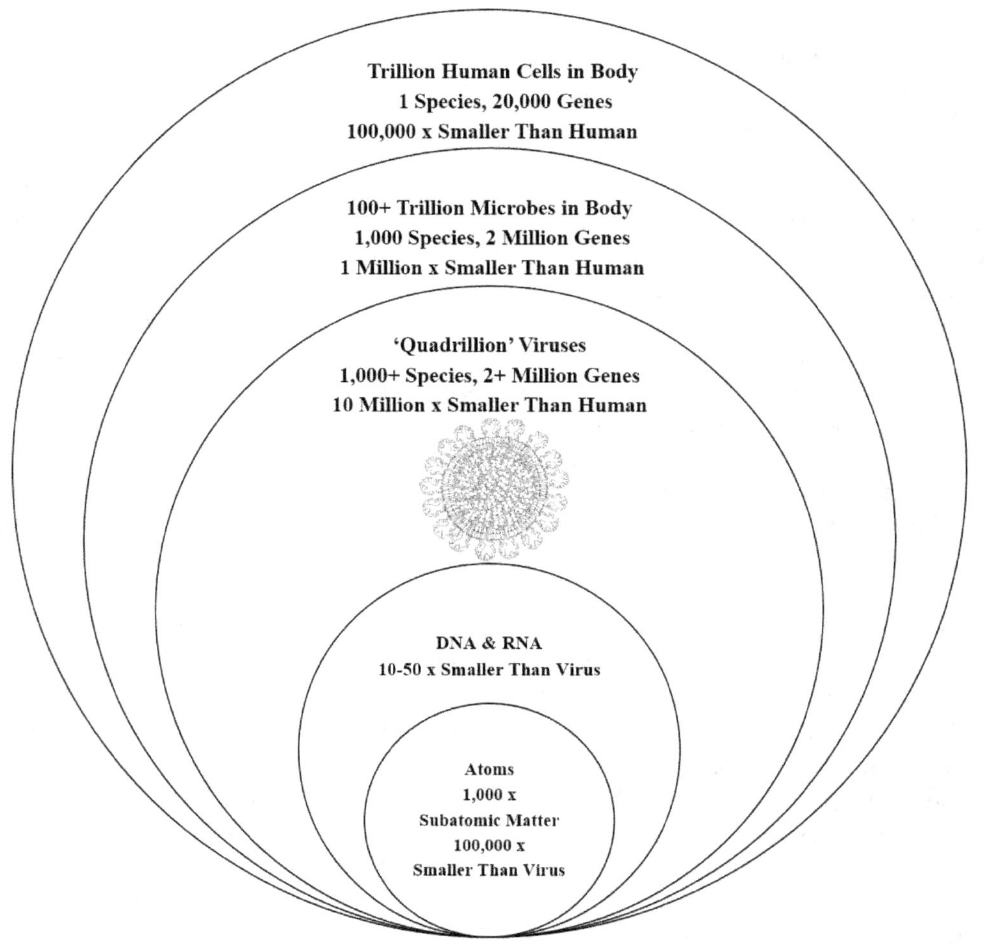

[b]D.S. Goodsell, M. Voigt, C. Zardecki, S.K. Burley. Integrative Illustration for Coronavirus Outreach. PLoS Biology, 2020; 18(8):e3000815. doi:10.1371/journal.pbio.3000815.

II. To Flatten The Curve
Epidemic Curves, Mitigation & PPE

Perception is strong and sight weak. In strategy, it is important to see distant things as if they were close and to take a distanced view of close things.

—The Book of Five Rings by Miyamoto Musashi
  Japanese Swordsman, Philosopher, Strategist & Samurai

Flattening the curve is COVID-19's 'coat of arms.' A diverse range of trusted sources from the New York Times to the New England Journal of Medicine herald the paramount role that flattening the curve plays in navigating the COVID-19 pandemic. Be that as it may, flattening the curve is neither a novel concept nor a novice pursuit. Epidemic curves, derived from series of data points in continuum, have been used to visualize outbreaks for centuries, from cholera in London 1854 to yellow fever in Angola 2016 and, of course, to COVID-19 in *World* 2019 to present.

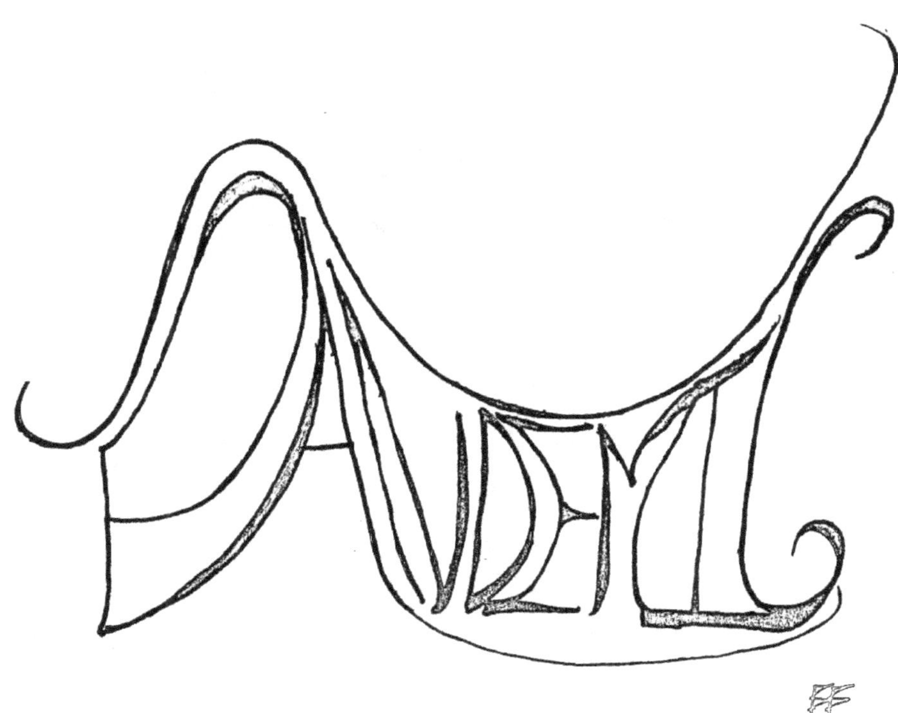

THE FIVE TYPES OF EPIDEMIC CURVES

So, let us start from the beginning with the basics: how an outbreak of an existing infectious agent works[6]. Classically, forces of nature forge the path for the ebb and flow of an infectious agent that is *endemic*, meaning exists in a population, at a low prevalence (total number of cases) and low incidence (total number of new cases). Then, by random chance or manmade manipulation, the natural history of the infectious agent changes. A perfect storm disrupts nature's system of checks and balances providing the infectious agent an opportunity to 'spike' the primordial soup to survive, thrive, and conquer unabated. The moment the mortal infectious agent peaks, it inevitably experiences an exaggerated decline followed by a reset back to its regularly scheduled programming in nature.

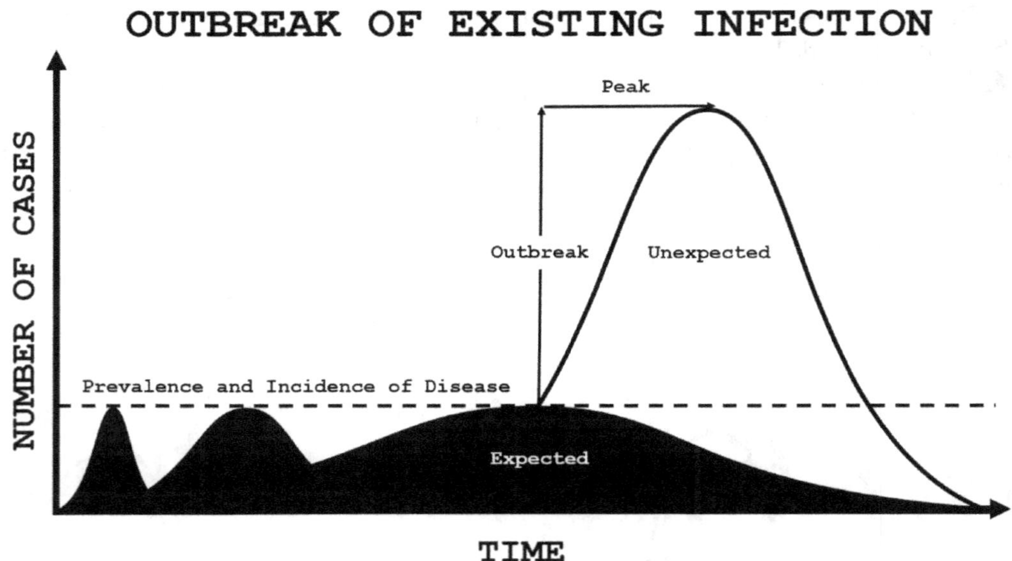

Next, we will take a deep dive into the different types of outbreaks. First, let us think of COVID-19 as a point source outbreak[6]. In this scenario, a common source (feel free to pick your COVID-19 'origins' camp, conspiracy, or school of thought) transmits an infection to others and the cycle of exposure, transmission, disease, death, or recovery occurs over a short period of time, typically one incubation period (life cycle of the infectious agent in the host body). Examples of point source outbreaks have historically been hepatitis A and other diarrheal illnesses in contaminated foods or food handlers.

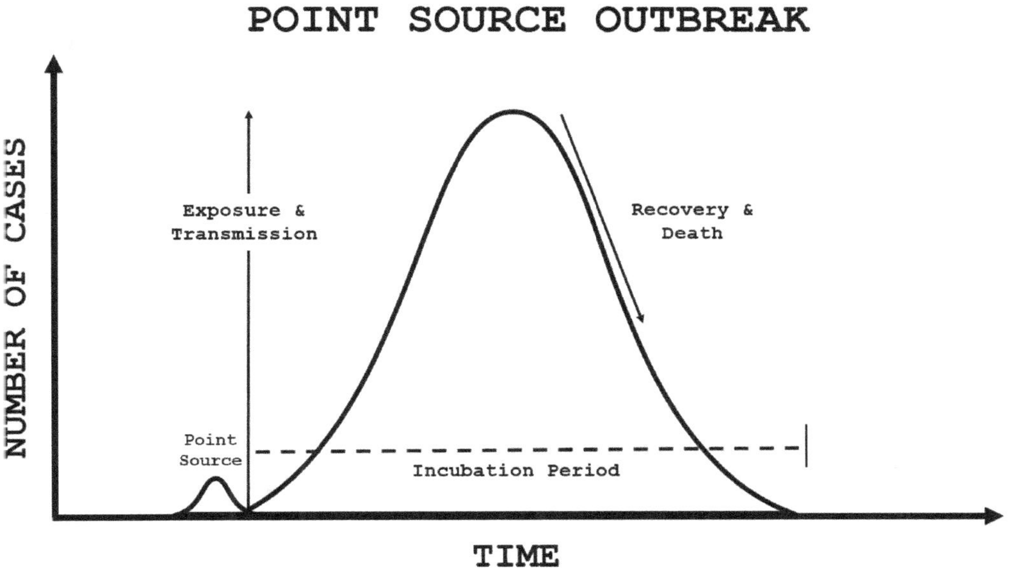

Now, let us think of COVID-19 as a continuous common source outbreak[6]. Here, cases peak and fall like point source outbreaks but not within a single incubation period because of ongoing sources of infection. A sharp decline from the peak signifies the main source of infection has been handled, whereas a gradual decline means the infection has run its course by fending off pockets of infection naturally or by means of mitigation strategies (public health strategies to flatten the curve). Outbreaks like cholera in the 1850s had this pattern because of ongoing infection from a common sewage source in pre-plumbing America.

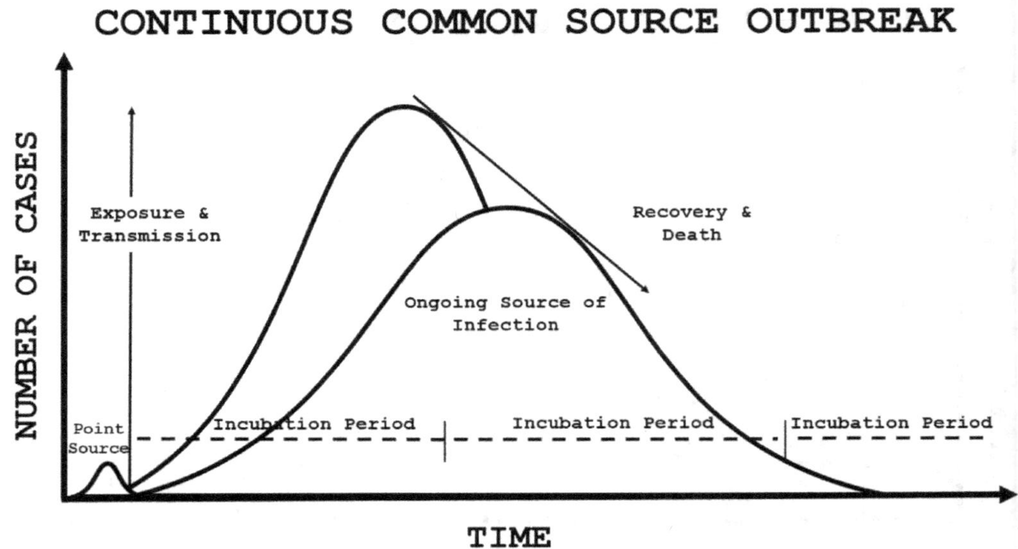

Next, let us think of COVID-19 as a propagated source outbreak[6], like pre-vaccine measles outbreaks in the 1950s and 1960s, that begins with a single index case that then spreads from person-to-person. Those initially infected make up the first wave who then infect another group of people who become the second wave. In this model, transmission is person-to-person rather than from a common source. There are a series of larger peaks at least one incubation period apart.

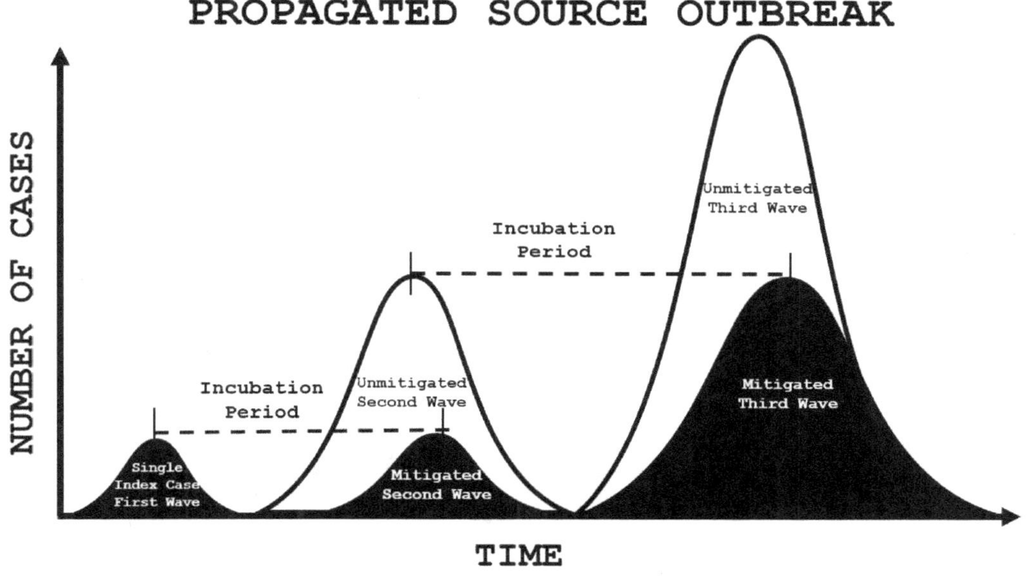

And finally, there is a rare model: the intermittent source outbreak[6]. It more commonly manifests in the wild, mainly in non-human, animal-to-animal contact following the touch-and-go synergistic or antagonistic interactions in nature. Aside from tribal communities or niche societies, it is not a pattern commonly seen in human outbreaks.

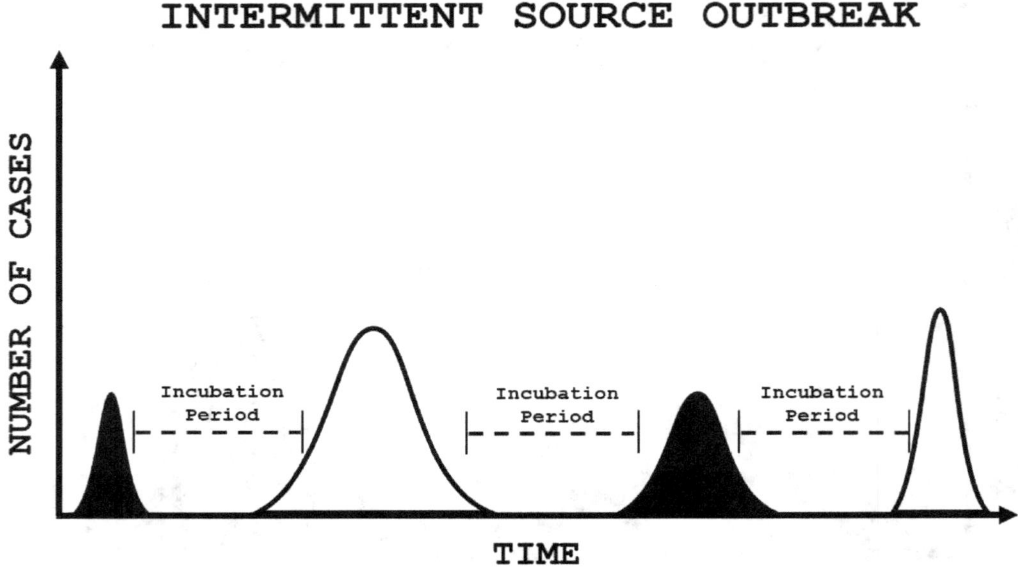

COVID-19 EPIDEMIOLOGY

COVID-19 is a mixed source outbreak turned pandemic. It is mainly a hybrid of point source, continuous common source, and propagated source outbreaks that has taken on different forms at different points in time. The first index case(s) in Wuhan, COVID-19's first *presumed* epicenter, prompted the first wave. This microcosm acted as a self-limited point source outbreak[7]. But, at the same time as a cohort of people was infected from a single source, other cohorts were infected from multiple sources and person-to-person transmission. Transmission spread from province to province in China in continuous common source and propagated outbreak patterns with ongoing sources of infection[8]. As mitigation strategies were implemented, transmission started to follow a point source outbreak pattern. As COVID-19's country of origin experienced a downward trend of infection, other countries experienced their first wave of this mounting epidemic. Countries like Italy, with a large older demographic, that were blind-sided by COVID-19, were similarly hit by a continuous common source outbreak. Italy served as martyr and maverick with regards to lives lost and lessons learned, respectively[9].

Some countries took heed to morbid messages more than others. Countries unprepared for the current pandemic, like the US, initially experienced a continuous common source outbreak. Early on, uncontrolled transmission led to anonymous, ongoing sources of infection[10]. Delayed mitigation strategies prolonged the downward trend. And now, the evaluation of how tactical reopening and relaxation of mitigation strategies is being judged in real time. Rather than learn from mistakes made during the first wave of COVID-19 in states hit the hardest like New York and New Jersey, several states initially unscathed by high rates of infection are just *now* experiencing rising numbers. Oddly enough, infection patterns are mimicking the intermittent source outbreak typically seen in animal, tribal, and niche populations. Spikes seem to correlate with events ranging from predictable cultural gatherings to eager masses congregating for re-opening of social institutions or engagement in social revolt. Fortunately, remnant mitigation strategies carried over from the first wave have provided some control over a potentially calamitous situation.

For countries more prepared for the pandemic that either enforced early mitigation strategies and/or controlled transmission (South Korea[11], Iceland[12], New Zealand[13], Norway[14], Denmark[15], Germany[16], Taiwan[17], and others), their people experienced a pseudo-point source outbreak. Unfortunately, re-opening in countries both prepared and unprepared for COVID-19 did not work out as intended. Few things in nature ever do.

With many countries in the developing world now reaching catastrophic numbers, countries in the developed world with previously low rates of infection and death are experiencing a modest to significant rise in cases. And unfortunately, the intended use of the 'immunity passport' and 'risk-free certificate' conferred by the practice of herd immunity is not as robust as hypothesized[18]. So please, <u>do not throw a COVID party</u>. Based on conservative epidemiological projections, if approximately 30% of a population is infected with a virus like SARS-CoV-2 and presumably develops antibodies, this halts the transmission of the virus to the population at large, a concept known as herd immunity. However, a recent study in Sweden, a prototype of herd immunity practices, demonstrated that less than 10% of people in Stockholm had antibodies as of late April 2020[19]. This too must be taken with a grain of salt. Antibodies take time to develop, permanence of antibodies is questionable, and testing has varying degrees of false negative and false positive rates. Officials report that 1 in 5 or 20% of people are predicted to have antibodies, but these results are not yet substantiated. And so, as the COVID-19 pandemic curve depicts, our global and national trajectories are uncertain[20].

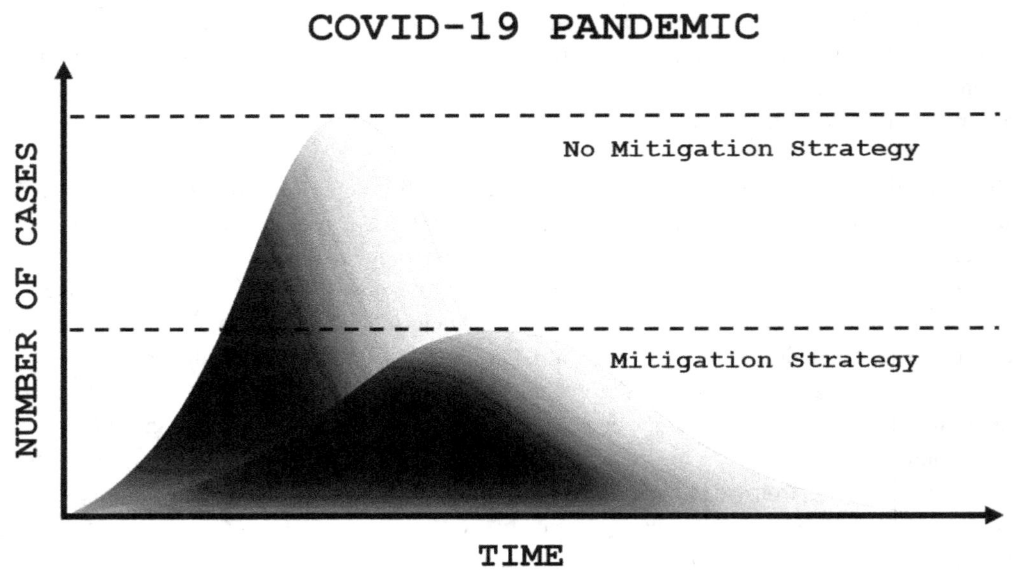

As this saga unravels, it exposes an important reality. Although leaders in the field and powers that be have tremendous influence over us, they are also vulnerable to the same mistakes that all of us face, except on a bigger stage. Keep this in mind as you read on. Together, if we become a more empowered people who are more knowledgeable about the pandemic at hand, we will burn the iron curtain needed to influence leaders and those in power to work harder for us in the spirit of transparency, goodwill, and respect.

PPE & MITIGATION

One can argue that personal protective equipment, or PPE, is unfairly distributed. With the post-quarantine, low-risk person at the grocery store unnecessarily sporting a gas mask and the frontline doctor or nurse scavenging the hospital for PPE before entering the room of a COVID-19 ICU patient, this is hard to refute. Asymptomatic carriers should wear a mask, but…*wait for it*…healthy contacts may not need to wear a mask[21,22] (in a perfect world, which ours certainly is not). Continuous micro-exposure to environmental pathogens is *healthy* for the healthy contact. The risk of SARS-CoV-2 transmission from a socially distanced, masked asymptomatic carrier to an unmasked healthy contact is indeed very low. The unfortunate reality is that testing is not widely available and available testing has significant false negative rates conferring a false sense of security. Moreover, the concept of the 'healthy contact' is misleading since people with a healthy-appearing phenotype, may have a vulnerable genotype and be none the wiser. And, it goes without saying, a symptomatic COVID-19 positive person should self-quarantine and high-risk people should abide by the most stringent of precautions on their own accord. But, how about the rest of us? In light of the circumstances, it appears safer for the asymptomatic carrier and healthy contact to *both* be masked. But, even these practices have fine print disclaimers with regards to sanitary mishaps and inconsistency outweighing practical benefit. At the very least, this 'anti-panic' rationale should alleviate some anxieties that have made presumably healthy contacts reluctant to help their fellow humans and be *humane*. Alas, common sense prevails again.

Unfortunately, as an educated citizen you carry the burden of recognizing that common sense is *not* common, and COVID-19 has certainly branded this rule and upped the ante on societal breakdown. Exaggerated social distancing in one location and non-existent social distancing '6 feet away' makes a large scale focus on interstate differences seem beside the point. Political trolling is puppeteering policy, industry, and 'herding' sheep mentality. In playing devil's advocate, people holding on to their 'constitutional rights,' hoarding, or being drawn to conspiracies as a means of making sense of the world are being force-fed misinformation, in lieu of a clear understanding of how bad things can *really* be, just like the rest of us. They just have different coping mechanisms.

Although solutions in a pandemic are best put to the test in real-time, the concept of a nationally-led system of state-specific 'experts' who formulate healthcare and socioeconomic policies to facilitate decision-making and re-opening strategies is most likely to align with 'the people' and *actually* happen, with a more manageable degree of protest. And perhaps, no other element of pandemic management unmasks a poorly built infrastructure more than the next matter at hand: testing.

Your Mask is Not a Wonderwall. Below is a version of a popular online graphic showing the risk of SARS-CoV-2 transmission between the masked and unmasked asymptomatic carrier and healthy contact. These numbers are *not* representative of current scientific evidence or literature. However, the rationale of the overall trend is sound. As mentioned above, the masked asymptomatic carrier mitigates risk of transmission exponentially. On the other hand, hubris aside, unmasked 'healthy contacts' cannot be sure of their invulnerability making the use of a mask imperative.

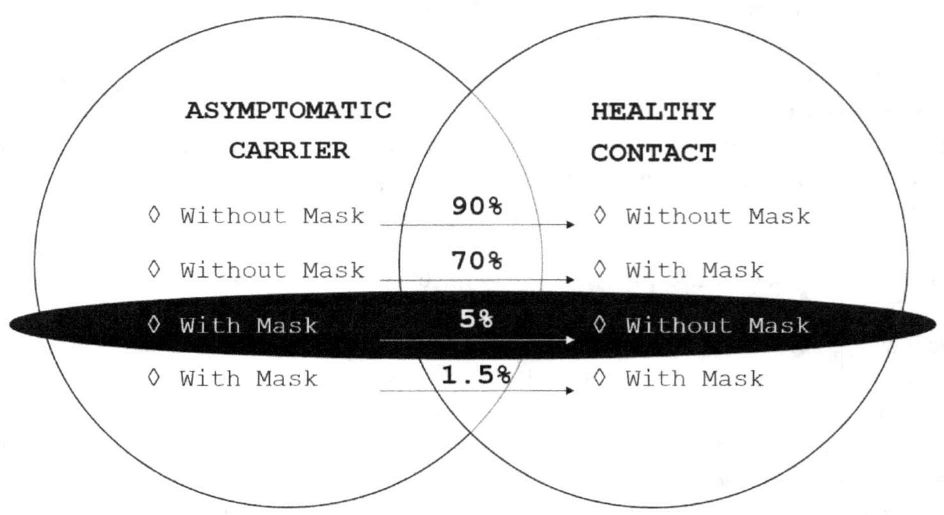

The Mitigation Strategy Checklist. You may have experienced the following mitigation 'matrix glitches.' Feel free to grade each type of governmental response as excellent, fair, or poor. Please also write in your own ideas, and refer to this chart as you read on.

Mitigation Strategy	Excellent	Fair	Poor
Common Sense Social Distancing			
Self-Quarantining for Symptomatic People			
Protection of High-Risk Groups			
Utilization of Essential Workers			
Outcomes of Herd Immunity Approaches			
Personal Protective Equipment			
Early, Accurate, Reliable, and Accessible Testing			
Ventilator and Resource Allocation			
State-Specific 'Expert' Leaders			
Research and Innovation			
Fair Market Pricing			
Addressing Mental Health Impact			
Management of Socioeconomic Fallout			

III. Gatekeeper Defense

Antibodies, Ace, Reinfection & Bad Tests

It must be remembered that there is nothing more difficult to plan, more doubtful of success, nor more dangerous to manage than a new system. For the initiator has the enmity of all who would profit by the preservation of the old institution and merely lukewarm defenders in those who gain by the new ones.

—The Prince by Niccolò Machiavelli
  Italian Renaissance Diplomat & Father of Political Science Philosophy

The fate of an outbreak, epidemic, or pandemic is at the mercy of its host population's strongest defense, which in the case of COVID-19 has been appointed as 'The Antibody.' As we will see, the designated omnipotence of the COVID-19 antibody should rightfully be called into question. On the other hand, the fate of the individual host is largely dependent on the dual gatekeeper roles of angiotensin-converting enzyme, or ACE, and spike protein that serve as SARS-CoV-2's dark horse and Achilles heel. And so, with projections uncertain, a cryptic defense, and a duplicitous gatekeeper, the rapid evolution of COVID-19 continues to threaten our ability to adapt.

Antibodies 101

Antibodies are known as immunoglobulins. They are made by plasma cells, a type of immune system 'B' cell, and are found in the *plasma* (clear, non-bloody) part of blood. A healthy immune system uses antibodies to neutralize pathogenic viruses. Antibodies recognize signature markings on viruses called antigens. In the case of vaccines (to be discussed properly), antigens are proteins identical or near identical to the pathogen intended to fool the immune system's frontline defense. Antigens bind to antibodies and tag pathogens for destruction. Pathogens are destroyed directly by blocking what viruses need to invade and survive or via other parts of the immune system (Pac Man-like macrophages). There are two types of B cells. Some are antibody factories (plasma cells) and others are experienced first responders (memory cells) that remember the plan of attack if a second wave of intruders manages to breach enhanced post-first invasion security. There are different types of antibodies designated as 'Ig' (short for immunoglobulin) followed by a letter. Pathogenic bacteria and other microbes are similarly neutralized by the immune system.

Role of the Antibody in Fighting a Pathogenic Virus	
IgM	Fights pathogens early on before enough IgG is produced. Measured in some SARS-CoV-2 antibody tests.
IgG	The major player in immunity that takes <u>weeks</u> or more to build up, provides long-lasting immunity, and crosses the placenta to give immunity to the fetus. Main antibody type measured in SARS-CoV-2 antibody testing.
IgA	Found in mucous, guts, respiratory tract, genitals, saliva, tears, and breast milk. Works on the frontlines to prevent colonization and transmission, or a virus from going *viral*. Rarely, if ever, measured in SARS-CoV-2 antibody testing.
IgE	Does not play a significant role in viral infections. An important part of the allergic response and protective against parasitic worms.
IgD	Does not play a known role in infection.

Most people who have had COVID-19 have antibodies. But, having antibodies is *not* the same as having immunity to the virus, and oftentimes antibodies quickly dissipate making 'immunity' a flash in the pan[23]. In my personal experience and those of other high-exposure frontline healthcare workers, most of us tested negative for active infection and antibodies after months of exposure and breaches in PPE. On the other hand, less exposed healthcare workers, some of whom were in the community and working remotely during the pandemic, tested positive for active or past infection. Even high-exposure frontline healthcare workers who displayed pathognomonic signs and symptoms of COVID-19, some of whom required hospitalization, perplexedly tested 'negative' for active and past infection. In non-COVID-19 medicine, a number of diseases are primarily a 'clinical diagnosis' while specific tests serve a subordinate role to *support* the clinical diagnosis. Similarly, and so long as we are able to separate ourselves from the 'everything-is-COVID-19' mentality, it may be reasonable to diagnosis COVID-19 clinically and not rely so heavily on imperfect testing.

The relationship between degree of exposure, likelihood of infection, and timing of testing is no doubt very complex. For now, there is limited evidence that people who have recovered from COVID-19 and have antibodies are protected from a second infection. People who assume they are immune to a second infection because they have received a positive qualitative (yes/no, positive/negative, present/absent) antibody test result may become asymptomatic carriers and ignore public health mitigation strategies risking transmission to others[24]. This false sense of security is why it is important to know the raw number, or *quantitative* level, of antibodies as opposed to a qualitative result. Unfortunately, most commercially available tests are qualitative and do not distinguish between IgG or IgM. And of course, testing almost never measures the unassuming, yet essential worker of the immune system: IgA.

NATURAL BORN KILLERS

Although not as coveted as IgG and IgM, IgA is essential. In fact, people with genetic disorders that prevent them for producing IgA are highly susceptible to a myriad of infections and disease. However, even in healthy populations, some people produce more IgA than others. This is one reason why some people are more prone to respiratory infections and sensitive to foreign gastrointestinal exposures as compared to their 'iron stomach' counterparts.

In the respiratory tract, IgA in the saliva and mucous blocks pathogen entry and manipulates the inflammatory response. Theoretically, in SARS-CoV-2, people with significantly higher levels of IgA may be less likely to 'catch' the virus because it is unable to pass the IgA-rich mucous barrier to colonize and invade. In turn, they are also less likely to transmit the virus after exposure. IgA works similarly in tears and eye infection. In the gut, IgA is induced by resident 'good' microbes. IgA is able to partially neutralize pathogens and exotoxins produced by infectious agents such as salmonella and E. coli. In breast milk, IgA plays a role in prevention of infection in the infant albeit without the lasting immunity of IgG. And unfortunately, in the genitals IgA is less predominant than IgG, which makes transmission of sexually transmitted diseases easier since IgG takes time to build its line of defense against its target pathogen.

BAD TESTS ARE INSENSITIVE

Laboratories perform SARS-CoV-2 antibody testing and nasal and/or oral swab testing for active infection with varying degrees of accuracy and reliability[25,26]. The gold standard for measuring test quality is sensitivity and specificity. A test that is 99% sensitive means it detects an infection or disease if *present* 99% of the time. A test that is 75% sensitive means it detects an infection or disease if present 75% of the time leaving 25% of the infected or diseased population with a false sense of security. A test that is 99% specific means it rules out infection or disease if *absent* 99% of the time. A test that is 75% specific means that it rules out an infection or disease if absent 75% of the time leaving 25% of the healthy population with unwarranted concern.

Sensitivity	
What is the proportion of people **with** an infection or disease who are accurately identified as having the infection or disease, or true positive rate?	
True Positives: Number of sick people who test positive. False Negatives: Number of sick people who test negative.	Sensitivity = $\dfrac{\text{True Positives}}{\text{True Positives} + \text{False Negatives}}$

Specificity
What is the proportion of people **without** an infection or disease who are accurately identified as not having the infection or disease, or true negative rate?

True Negatives: Number of healthy people who test negative. False Positives: Number of healthy people who test positive.	Specificity= $\dfrac{\text{True Negatives}}{\text{True Negatives} + \text{False Positives}}$

Screening tests such as home pregnancy tests typically have a very high sensitivity to rule out false negatives. Confirmation tests after a screening test for infections such as HIV typically have very high specificity to rule out false positives. In the case of a pandemic from a novel infection, circumstances are far from controlled. At the onslaught of COVID-19, a flurry of 'viral load' testing became available. In infectious agents that primarily spread via the respiratory route, screening tests that use nasal and/or oral samples to measure viral load are standard. Although a subset of available tests has high sensitivity, many tests have lower sensitivity, meaning some people who have signs and symptoms of infection test negative. In the hospital, if there is high suspicion that a person has the infection or disease and only a low sensitivity test is available, the test is often repeated 2 or even 3 times to increased its combined sensitivity. In the community, the heterogeneity of test sensitivity taints epidemiological efforts to identify the number of 'true positive' cases. Given the gastrointestinal symptoms people with COVID-19 often present with and the likelihood that transmission is also via the fecal-oral route (or at the very least viral shedding continues longer in feces than nasal and/or oral secretions), fecal testing is under-utilized and, to our detriment, sparingly available[27].

A number of antibody blood tests are susceptible to the same limitations of low sensitivity and specificity. Moreover, timing of antibody testing and type of antibodies tested are important given mounting IgM and delayed IgG responses early in the disease course. In fact, some antibody tests have increased time-dependent sensitivity, meaning, for example, they are 60% sensitive Day 0, 75% sensitive Day 7, and 90% sensitive Day 14 post-exposure. And as we now know, the mere presence of antibodies does not equate to infection exclusivity.

ACE AT THE PERIMETER

SARS-CoV-2 and other coronaviruses like MERS-CoV and SARS-CoV invade human host cells with the help of receptors for angiotensin converting enzyme-2/angiotensin 1-7, herein referred to as ACE[28]. A receptor, or landing pad, aids and abets the infectious agent into its target cell. Enzymes are proteins made in the body that are in charge of powering a vital and specific function. ACE wears many hats, plays a principle role in nearly all aspects of COVID-19, and will be interjected at nauseam in this manifesto. ACE is found in the lungs (overproduced in smokers and chronic lung disease), kidneys, brain, heart, testicles, gastrointestinal system, mucous membranes, some immune cells, and endothelium (inner lining of the blood vessels). Some types of ACE promote all that is good (anti-cell death, anti-fibrosis, anti-blood vessel constriction, anti-clotting, anti-heart failure, anti-heart wall thickening, anti-plaque formation, anti-heart rhythm abnormalities, anti-endothelial dysfunction related to metabolic syndrome, et cetera), whereas others types of ACE do the polar opposite. Just as individual differences exist in IgA, people have genetic differences in ACE genes. This is a common phenomenon known as polymorphism literally meaning many (*poly-*) variants *(-morphism)*. There is early evidence that different ACE polymorphisms respond differently to some viruses[29], but no definitive associations can be made.

In contrast to the theoretical risk of increased viral colonization and transmission, the role of ACE in coronavirus infection in ameliorating acute lung injury and mitigating secondary injury to the heart and kidneys is well-studied[28]. Moreover, in an attempt to outsmart SARS-CoV-2 at its own game, experimental clinical trials of faux-ACE agents that bind to the virus to prevent colonization and invasion are currently underway. In addition, Spike, the protein on SARS-CoV-2 that enhances the ability of the virus to attach to the ACE receptor, is also a promising target for COVID-19 treatment and vaccine development[30].

THE HYPERTENSION CONTROVERSY

ACE is part of a larger piece of machinery in the body called the renin-angiotensin-aldosterone system, or simply RAAS. Medications for blood pressure, specifically, ACE-inhibitors and ARBs (angiotensin receptor blockers) like lisinopril and losartan, respectively, are commonly used in hypertension. ACE-inhibitors and ARBS are enemy antagonists to the RAAS system. Theoretically, stopping RAAS lets ACE run rampant and more ACE means more receptors for SARS-CoV-2, a higher viral load, and increased susceptibility. Therefore, there has been debate in the media and scientific community as to whether people with COVID-19 should generally consider stopping their ACE-inhibitor or ARB. Stopping these medications in high-risk people with heart failure, coronary heart disease, kidney problems, or heart attack is <u>not</u> recommended for people at risk for, being evaluated for, or with COVID-19.

In MERS-CoV, SARS-CoV, and SARS-CoV-2, preliminary studies show that a history of ACE-inhibitor or ARB use is not associated with increased severity of COVID-19 after adjusting for confounding variables[31,32]. At the extreme end of spectrum in the COVID-19 ICU, ACE-inhibitors and ARBs are stopped. But, this is *not* because of the aforementioned anecdotal concerns. Rather, most home medications that are futile, counterproductive, or potentially harmful are generally stopped in critically ill patients, who are often faced with paradoxical problems in a parallel universe of their regular lives. In line with the enigmatic features of COVID-19, our next venture delves into its paradoxical effect on blood and the humors.

IV. THERE WILL BE BLOOD

BLOOD TYPE, CLOTS, SPIKE & ECMO

Your blood is in the war. In your arteries is the power to give men a second chance to live.

—*Vogue* (1943) by Edgar L. Jones on Segregation of Blood Supply During World War II
WWII Veteran, Merchant Seaman & Army Historian

Just like us, the intelligent contagion that survives a war relies on principles 'older-than-time' to guide its evolution. The four humors, first described by Hippocrates, is a modern-day scientific truth that embraced the commonality of everything greater than skin-deep, even in ancient times. Ironically, as far removed as evidence-based medicine presently is from the mystical and metaphysical, the humors were historically embraced by an eclectic range of people outside of the scientific bubble, from alchemist to enlightened artistic mastermind. Fast forward to COVID-19, where disharmony between the humors of blood (sanguine), plasma (phlegmatic), inflammation (choleric), and clotting factors (melancholic) still simply and elegantly describe the tactical and operational strategies of the microscopic enemy we have made in COVID-19.

BLOOD TYPE MATTERS

Viruses including SARS-CoV-2 are influenced by blood type[33] and change important factors in how blood clots[34]. There are four main blood types. Type A blood has A antigen on red blood cells and anti-B antibody in plasma, so type A blood cannot receive type B blood. Type B blood has B antigen on red blood cells and anti-A antibody in plasma, so type B blood cannot receive type A blood. Type AB blood has AB antigen on red blood cells and no anti-A or anti-B antibodies, which makes people with type AB blood universal acceptors who can only donate to other type AB blood types. Type O blood type has no antigens on red blood cells and both anti-A and anti-B antibodies, which makes people with type O blood type universal donors who can only accept blood from other type O blood types.

Blood Type	Antigen	Antibody	Able to Donate To	Able to Accept From
A	A	Anti-B	A, AB	A, O
B	B	Anti-A	B, AB	B, O
AB	AB	—	AB	A, B, AB, O
O	—	Anti-A, Anti-B	A, B, AB, O	O

Coronaviruses such as SARS-CoV and, more recently, SARS-CoV-2 may share an association with type O blood and low infection rates, and type A blood and higher infection rates. The hypothesis behind this anomaly is that anti-A antibodies found on type O (and to a lesser extent on type B) blood prevents SARS-CoV-2 from binding to ACE[33]. Although current studies have several limitations, if well-designed studies in the future support these findings, then people with type A blood may need more 'high-tech' PPE for prevention, better surveillance and aggressive treatment for COVID-19, and blood type testing may become a standard part of COVID-19 management.

BLOOD *IS* THICKER

As a stroke physician, I treat neurological consequences of hypercoagulable (pro-clotting) states from diseases such as cancer that make the blood hyper-viscous (extra thick), autoimmune disorders like lupus that usurp the inflammatory cascade, and sickle cell disease that causes the blood to *sickle*, or stick together. 'Thicker' blood gets lodged into relatively small blood vessels like clogged pipes in plumbing. This leads to blockages in the brain's arteries (strokes) or veins (sinus thromboses), lungs (pulmonary emboli), legs (deep vein thromboses), et cetera.

So, how do severe forms of COVID-19 and other viral diseases create a hypercoagulable state that, as it turns out, is a hallmark of non-survivors? ACE, the receptor for SARS-CoV-2, lines the endothelium inside of blood vessels. Viral pathogens influence the behavior of blood vessels via numerous substances such as tissue factor creating a cascade of chaos that disrupts homeostasis, or balance, between pro-clotting and anti-clotting factors in the body. Many pathogens disrupt homeostasis, causing blood to be too thin and prone to hemorrhage or bleeding (coagulopathic) or hypercoagulable. The worst-case scenario is a disease process known as disseminated intravascular coagulation, or DIC. In DIC, highly virulent pathogens enter the bloodstream leading to a refractory consumption of clotting factors, simultaneous hemorrhage and thrombosis (clotting), and the poorest prognosis.

Many infectious agents affect blood clotting, not just SARS-CoV-2. Ebola is associated with hemorrhage, CMV with thrombosis, and herpes zoster with both. HIV, EBV (aka mono, the 'kissing disease'), parvovirus B19, hepatitis, hantavirus, Marburg virus, and Dengue are just on the shortlist of culprits. But, do *not* freak out. Just as in COVID-19, generally only people with a weakened immune system or other significant risk factors are at risk for these serious complications.

For people who do develop severe COVID-19, there is evidence that early anticoagulation meaning putting patients on blood thinners, or anti-coagulation, at a higher dose than would normally be used for prevention of blood clots in the hospital, may be beneficial. Interestingly anti-coagulation may also abate infectivity of SARS-CoV-2. As you know, ACE is activated by Spike protein and promotes infectivity. It just so happens that Spike is activated by key clotting factors, which was studied during the SARS epidemic years ago[35]. And so, it is hypothesized that anti-coagulation may limit SARS-CoV-2 replication by inactivating Spike thereby indirectly reducing ACE activity. Albeit promising, this hypothesis requires further investigation. Early evidence from human clinical trials also demonstrates that anti-coagulants have a formidable anti-inflammatory effect, most notably on interleukin-6 (IL-6)[36], which we will soon discover is one of the key players in the cytokine storm.

But please, steer clear of herbal supplements that claim to cleanse or thin the blood. Also, it is not recommended that people outside of a hospital or clinical trial setting start taking blood thinners. Rather, simple lifestyle changes such as staying *very* well hydrated and physically active make all the difference. Admittedly, prior to my residency and fellowship training, I thought staying hydrated and exercising was a generic recommendation, but I have seen dehydration and immobility cause stroke and other neurovascular conditions by means of festering stagnancy of blood that makes one prone to clotting.

HAIL MARY —ECMO

In patients who are refractory to maximal protective ventilator and positioning strategies, paralyzing (on purpose, of course), and optimization of fluid balance, a Hail Mary intervention known as ECMO may be an option. ECMO stands for extracorporeal membrane oxygenation. It is a form of extra-corpeal (outside the living body, literally) life support that does the work of the lungs and heart outside of the body. Here is how:

◊ First, tubing is placed in a large vein such as the femoral vein in the crease of the groin.
◊ Second, low oxygen blood in the body travels through tubing to a 'pump' outside the body that mimics the heart.
◊ Third, blood travels from the 'pump' to an 'oxygenator' outside the body that mimics the lungs and is attached to a heating/cooling system.
◊ Fourth, normal, oxygen-rich blood travels back through tubing into the body via another large vein or the main artery of the body, the aorta.

Because of the risks ECMO poses, general pre-COVID-19 guidelines have been developed to limit its use[37]. Patients should be on the ventilator for less than 7 days, be less than 65 years old, be in critical condition, and meet the following criteria clinically and arterial blood gas, or ABG:

◊ Low oxygen levels in the lungs despite artificial supply of oxygen through the breathing tube and ventilator.
◊ High carbon dioxide levels in the lungs secondary to poor ventilation and gas exchange.
◊ High lung pressures as measured on the ventilator associated with increased risk of lung injury, or barotrauma.
◊ Low oxygen levels in the blood indicating poor perfusion of blood, glucose, oxygen, and nutrients to different organs.

◊ High acid levels in the blood measured via bicarbonate signifying marked oxygen deprivation requiring the organs to undergo anaerobic (without oxygen) metabolism.

There is some evidence that (vein-to-vein) ECMO reduces high lung pressures, risk of lung trauma, or barotrauma (think of a pressure *baro*meter), and reduces inflammation in the lungs and body[38,39]. If a virus causes infection or inflammation of the heart, heart failure, or shock, then vein-to-artery ECMO is an option. There are even fancier, hybrid versions of ECMO, all of which share a very high-risk profile similar to traditional ECMO.

We will investigate the cytokine storm next chapter but suffice it to say, from the perspective of blood vessels, the cytokine storm renders blood vessels paralyzed and in a state of shock, whereby they are unable to meaningfully constrict, dilate, or pump blood throughout the body. Stagnant blood leads not only to blood clots but also to edema (swelling), oxygen deprivation, and death of endothelial cells lining the inside of blood vessels. In one sense, ECMO circuits eliminate pro-clotting and pro-inflammatory elements by irreversibly binding them to surface coating material within its machinery. In another sense, ECMO, by way of blood cells being exposed to a foreign system and shear stress, sets off pro-clotting and pro-inflammatory states that augment the cytokine storm. ECMO also inadvertently causes a deficiency in an important anti-inflammatory clotting factor: anti-thrombin. This further exacerbates the pro-inflammatory state in which critically ill COVID-19 patients already find themselves.

As we learned from our discussion of DIC, severe forms of COVID-19 and other viral diseases may cause a simultaneous clotting and bleeding state. A bleeding state is often precipitated by low platelets, or thrombocytopenia. And unfortunately, ECMO is associated with low platelets. However, it is a chicken or egg catch-22. Low platelets may be caused by ECMO itself or be an incidental finding given the severity of disease in patients who ultimately meet criteria for ECMO. One indirect benefit of ECMO, by no merit if its own, is the need for anti-coagulation while on ECMO to prevent blood clots. As discussed earlier, anti-coagulants have benefits in mitigating the pro-clotting and pro-inflammatory states in severe COVID-19 patients. It is also important to keep in mind that some anti-coagulants such as heparin, which is highly effective and reversible, is also rarely associated with low platelets secondary to an autoimmune reaction known as heparin-induced thrombocytopenia, or HIT. These HIT antibodies can be measured in the blood when there is a high suspicion.

Results of ECMO in COVID-19 are mixed[37]. Regardless, the FDA has approved and WHO and CDC have recommended the use of ECMO for the aforementioned indications in COVID-19[40]. However, given ECMO's high risk versus benefit profile, the inexperience of most centers with ECMO, scare resources during a pandemic in high-income countries, and limited to no availability in low- and middle-income countries, many ECMO specialists warn against the widespread use of ECMO on the frontlines[41].

For patients and physicians less inclined to 'ride the lightning,' there are more conservative ways to improve oxygen delivery and efficiency in the body. Transfusion of normal, well-oxygenated blood[42], medications to increase a person's own ability to make blood cells such as erythropoietin[43], or medications like cilostazol and sildenafil[44] that help existing blood cells delivery oxygen more efficiency may be used. The latter are members of a family of medications called phosphodiesterase inhibitors that optimize oxygen delivery to their target organ and are traditionally used for multiple indications including poor circulation in the legs (peripheral vascular disease) and penis ('vascular' erectile dysfunction). Some neurovascular specialists even use cilostazol for rare brain conditions such as moyamoya to increase oxygen delivery to the brain. Although ECMO may seem like a double-edged sword, perhaps the most compelling thing to remember about ECMO is that it does _not_ compromise antibody-based treatments including convalescent plasma, IV immunoglobulins, or tocilizumab, which would otherwise deter even the most gung-ho patients, families, and physicians.

V. I Am The Storm

Cytokine Storming & Covid-19 Biomarkers

Chaos was the law of nature; order was the dream of man.

—Henry Adams
Political Journalist Influenced by Civil War Diplomacy & Descendent of Two US Presidents

For decades, trending diets, fad detox programs, and hyped-up anti-aging products have ridden the coattails of the anti-inflammatory movement with promises of reversing the unattractive physical consequences of cumulative, microscopic damages over a lifetime…all by following a few simple steps. In reality, the organized chaos housed within the walls of the healthy human subject is not amendable to a 'steps 1 thru 3' approach or generic assembly line of well-marketed lotions and potions. At the opposite end of the spectrum, in the critically ill patient, organized chaos loses its nerve and falls into a state of natural lawlessness, where the line between the laws of nature and the unnatural are blurred. Firsthand accounts from doctors all around the world of the fulminant course of twists and turns 'no one has ever seen before' in the sickest of the sick with COVID-19 are largely attributable to the ferocious capacity of inflammation at its most infamous: the Cytokine Storm.

The cytokine storm

The cytokine storm is not a novel concept. It represents the zenith of macroscopic havoc a microscopic pro-inflammatory pathogen can ravage on the human body in its most vulnerable condition. Cytokine storming is triggered by both exogenous (foreign infection or severe injury) or endogenous (highly dysfunctional *auto*immune system) exposures.

In the media, the cytokine storm wears the COVID-19 scarlet letter for 'betraying the immune system of the young[45].' Albeit dramatic, it is true that the young immune system is more active and may *over*react more so than that of older people. Even within the same individual, an autoimmune disease that comes to fruition in youth may become dormant with age and immunosenescence, or senility of the immune system.

A cytokine is a substance made by the immune system that has a domino effect either for or against a particular process that is intended, as a whole, to create a balanced homeostatic environment. In a cytokine storm, homeostasis is compromised and there is an overproduction of pro-inflammatory cytokines. If the target is unable to weather the cytokine storm, then it becomes bigger, stronger, and equipped to invade and conquer a larger territory. People with a protoplasm more susceptible to COVID-19 experience this very exaggerated, aggressive, and refractory inflammatory response largely responsible for critical illness, multisystem organ failure, shock, and death[46].

Old and new therapeutics proposed to target overactive cytokines in COVID-19 do so via anti-inflammatory and/or immunomodulatory (immune system modulation or manipulation) properties. But, the strongest immunomodulator that markedly suppresses the immune system will inevitably cause harm. By figuratively putting the immune response out to pasture, the body's own immuno-inflammatory response grows inept at clearing dead pathogens from the body. This leaves the human host in the awkward and dangerous position of having defeated the enemy whilst having nowhere to hide except behind a mounting number of 'viral bodies.' This can have a paradoxical effect leading to yet another, even more powerful wave of cytokine storming.

This is yet another example highlighting the importance of *balance* and understanding that nothing is simply black and white within the human body. Unfortunately, the media and popular science often portray observations in black and white and label findings as cause-and-effect rather than taking a deeper (more challenging and less flashy dive) into the confounders of misleading associations. For example, when a news outlet reports a person with a compromised immune system at baseline chronically on a drug under investigation for the prevention or treatment of COVID-19 happens to contract COVID-19, it does *not* equate to ineffectiveness of the medication in another person without risk factors who is naive to the same medication. It is, therefore, imperative to take headlines intended to stir gossip and spark interest with a grain of salt, which you can only do effectually by reading between the lines.

BIOMARKERS ON PAR

Another division of key players in the cytokine storm are part of the coagulation, or pro- and anti-blood clotting, pathway. Thrombin is responsible for clot formation via activating platelets. Platelets are biomarkers of disease severity as well as indirect measures of safety and effectiveness of treatment. Thrombin also regulates inflammation via a family of factors known as peroxisome proliferator-activated receptors, or simply PPARs.

Alongside biomarkers like tissue factor, PPAR also becomes unhinged during the cytokine storm[47]. In the early phase, PPAR activation has been shown to limit viral load in influenza A[48], protect against myocarditis (heart inflammation) in the Coxsackie virus[49], and reduce leakage of lipopolysaccharides (toxic juice Nerf-gunned out of pathogens) in bacterial pneumonia[50]. However, in later phases, PPAR activation decreases overall survival and demonstrates pro-inflammatory, pro-oxidant, and pro-clotting properties. Well-established anti-coagulants, such as the anti-thrombin agent heparin and factor Xa inhibitor apixaban, may ameliorate disease progression and severity of COVID-19[51] for a multitude of reasons including an inhibitory effect on PPAR. As mentioned time and again, anti-coagulation is challenging in critical illness given the simultaneous propensity for bleeding and clotting, which is why anti-coagulation should only be used in a controlled environment. To facilitate safer usage of anti-coagulation in general, a growing number of anti-coagulants now have reversal agents[52].

THE COVID LAB

Most hospitals have developed COVID-19-specific labs to standardize the evaluation and treatment of COVID-19 patients within their institutions. These 'COVID-19 labs' are a set of inflammatory biomarkers, some of which are more specific to COVID-19 than others. In some cases, it is helpful to trend inflammatory markers in patients who test negative for active infection initially or test negative for active infection after treatment[53]. For SARS-CoV-2 positive patients in the thick of it, inflammatory markers are trended to assess the efficacy of a treatment, adjudicate the etiology of problems that complicate the clinical course, or determine prognosis. Part of this panel includes SARS-CoV-2 viral load testing for active infection and SARS-CoV-2 antibody testing for prior infection or exposure, and these tests were discussed earlier in the text.

Biomarkers indicative of cytokine storming if up-trending include but are not limited to: interleukin-6 (IL-6), high sensitivity C-reactive protein (CRP), ferritin, D-dimer, creatinine phosphokinase (CPK), lactate dehydrogenase (LDH), kidney and liver function tests, and coagulation factors or 'coags' including international normalized ratio (INR), prothrombin time (PT), and partial thromboplastin time (PTT). A biomarker suggestive of worsening cytokine storming if down trending is absolute lymphocyte count (ALC), which indicates suppression of the immune system. Some biomarkers such as glucose and platelets may fluctuate greatly during the clinical course, with either extreme raising concern. CD8 T cells, while low in peripheral blood, are highly concentrated in the lungs and perpetuate lung injury. Loss of albumin in the body and high protein in the urine are indirect biomarkers of systemic malfunction secondary to cytokine storming[46]. Another important biomarker in COVID-19 management is the QT interval, aka the root-cause behind all the hype on hydroxychloroquine, which we discuss next.

Biomarker	Up	Down	Mechanism
IL-6	X		Target of tocilizumab (IL-6 inhibitor)
CRP	X		High in chronic inflammatory conditions
Ferritin	X		High in anemia of chronic disease
D-dimer	X		High in acute pulmonary embolism
CPK	X		High in heart and skeletal muscle breakdown
LDH	X		High in low oxygen states
Renal Function	X		Blood urea nitrogen (BUN) and creatinine
Liver Function	X		Aspartate (AST)/alanine (ALT) aminotransferases and bilirubin
Coags	X		Evaluated with INR, PT, and PTT
Urine Protein	X		Loss of protein and nutrients in damaged kidneys
ALC		X	Low absolute lymphocyte count to fight infection
Albumin		X	Exodus of protein in circulation into soft tissue
CD8 T cells	X	X	Low in blood and high in injured lungs
Glucose	X	X	Extreme values associated with poor prognosis
Platelets	X	X	Extremes values associated with poor prognosis and bleeding

VI. WAR PROPOGANDA

THE MISEDUCATION OF QT & HYDROXYCHLOROQUINE

All the war-propaganda, all the screaming and lies and hatred, comes invariably from people who are not fighting.

—Homage to Catalonia by George Orwell
   Account of Experiences Soldiering for the Republican Army of the Spanish Civil War

Everything has a backstory if you look hard enough. But, life invariably gets in the way of taking a deep dive into every new and important subject, especially with the minute-to-minute coverage of COVID-19. For those of us too busy, too lazy, too keen on 'fighting the power,' or too frightened to question the status quo, information from a 'trusted' source, from your next door neighbor to your news feed, may seem like a more practical way hear the latest breaking news. However, this one-dimensional snapshot can influence your opinions of and reactions to other legitimate viewpoints, and worst of all, stop you from thinking for yourself. Such is the case with hydroxychloroquine.

THE ORPHAN DRUG

Approved for medical use in the US since 1955 and currently on the World Health Organization's List of Essential Medications[54], hydroxychloroquine (brand name Plaquenil) herein referred to as HCQ, is a controversial treatment in COVID-19. HCQ is not to be confused with chloroquine, which has a more severe side effect profile[55]. HCQ is FDA-approved for malaria prophylaxis and autoimmune diseases such as lupus and rheumatoid arthritis that commonly affect young women of childbearing age[56]. Although HCQ transfers into breast milk, studies demonstrate that it is safe in the pregnant mother, fetus, and child post-exposure[57,58]. HCQ is also low-cost and accessible, outside of the pandemic black hole vacuum.

As its use in autoimmune and infectious disease suggests, HCQ has anti-inflammatory, immunomodulatory, and anti-infective properties. One of the strongest hypotheses supporting the anti-infective properties of HCQ is its role as a 'zinc ionophore.' As we will discuss in later chapters, zinc has the potential to go DEFCON 0 on a virus. Zinc enters cells via special protein 'bouncers' that guard the zinc ionophore to ensure only zinc may enter. HCQ functions as a 'backdoor entrance' for zinc to increase the number of zinc molecules that enter the cell to kill the virus[59]. This explains why HCQ is more effective at preventing infection or in the early stages of infection where the processes of viral colonization, replication, and invasion are evolving.

QTC TV SUBLIMINAL MESSAGES

Adverse events related to HCQ are over-publicized, but they are indeed rare occurrences. HCQ may be associated with a heart rhythm abnormality, or cardiac arrhythmia, that is predicted in real-time by a progressively longer heart 'wave' on EKG or telemetry, known as the QT interval that is corrected for heart rate (QTc).

What is a QT interval? Think of the heart as an oddly built 4-bedroom house with 2 bedrooms upstairs and 2 downstairs. The upstairs rooms are the right and left atria. The downstairs rooms are the right and left ventricles. Blood from large veins in the body is pumped into the right atrium→right ventricle→lungs→left atrium→left ventricle→large artery (aorta)→body. The EKG is an electrical representation of the heart. The P wave indicates atrial contraction of blood. The QRS wave indicates ventricular contraction of blood. The ST segment is the time it takes for the ventricles to relax after contraction. The T and U waves represent 'rebooting' of the ventricles and specialized cells (Purkinje fibers) to prepare for the next contraction. And so, the QT interval is the time from contraction-to-contraction of the ventricles.

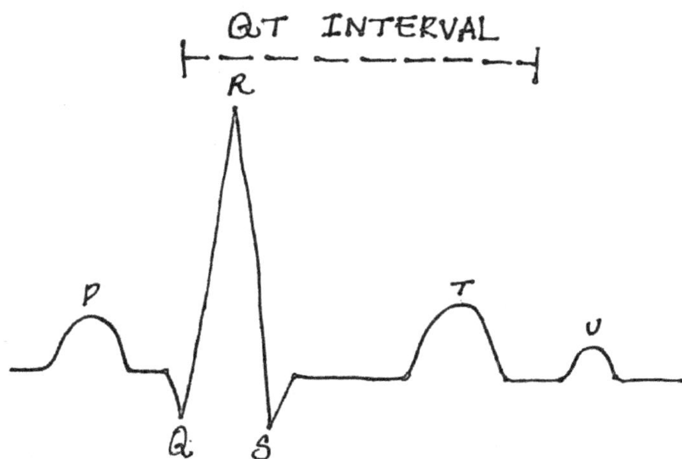

An abnormal QTc interval is >450 milliseconds in males and >470 milliseconds in females. If left untreated, a prolonged QTc may lead to an aberrant ventricular contraction rate and rhythm (ventricular tachycardia and fibrillation), torsade de pointes (a Kamikaze sinusoidal heart pattern), or sudden cardiac death. Over <u>100 medications</u> other than HCQ and many health conditions are associated with prolonged QTc interval including but not limited to: anti-nausea, anti-histamine, anti-fungal, antibiotic, antidepressant, antipsychotic, anti-arrhythmic, anti-organ rejection, anti-cancer, and diuretic medications as well as genetic disorders, hypothyroidism, anorexia, bulimia, low potassium, low calcium, and low magnesium levels. In HCQ, risk increases with concurrent use of other medications associated with QTc interval prolongation such as azithromycin (yes, Z-pack)[60]. Moreover, severe forms of COVID-19 may independently injure the heart muscle and precipitate rhythm abnormalities. Generally speaking, most significant side effects associated with HCQ are in chronic use for autoimmune diseases[61] and *not* short-term use for infectious disease prophylaxis. And as stated earlier, the incidence of COVID-19 in immunocompromised people on HCQ chronically does *not* equate to its ineffectiveness in other people without autoimmune disease who are naïve to the medication.

Although cardiac complications of HCQ are a prime focus, HCQ should also be used judiciously in other conditions. HCQ may lower blood glucose levels and is contraindicated in poorly controlled diabetes where blood sugar fluctuations are common. Caution must also be taken when HCQ is used along with medications such as digoxin that are metabolized by the liver since abnormally high or low levels of HCQ or its competitor may occur. Although HCQ is used for some dermatological conditions such as porphyria, it is contraindicated in psoriasis and may cause a paradoxical reaction. Concerns have also been raised regarding vision problems associated with HCQ. The potential for retinal damage is dose-dependent and very rare, even in people who take HCQ chronically[61]. It does not pose a significant risk for people on HCQ for days to weeks for infectious disease prophylaxis.

As of June 30, 2020, there were over 142 COVID-19 clinical trials studying HCQ alone. This is more than remdesivir, tocilizumab, and steroids combined[62]. The volume of data is overwhelming and study quality is highly variable. As such, HCQ clinical trials for safety and efficacy in treatment of COVID-19 are very mixed[63]. With regards to prevention of COVID-19 in frontline healthcare workers, studies are underway to evaluate safety and efficacy of HCQ in COVID-19 as pre-exposure prophylaxis[63,64]. Generalizability of these studies to the community will be challenging given that gauging community 'exposure' is difficult. An objective marker of 'pre-exposure' may well be interval testing regardless of symptoms to evaluate if people are negative for active infection and/or antibodies prior to initiation of HCQ as pre-exposure prophylaxis.

RETRACT, REDACT, RETREAT

The FDA recommends limiting HCQ use in COVID-19 to a hospital or clinical trial environment[65]. This FDA recommendation was largely based on a recent study published in a high impact medical journal that suggested HCQ is associated with cardiac arrhythmia and prolonged QTc interval in COVID-19. Soon after publication, the article was retracted because the sponsoring organization declined to share the study dataset, client contracts, and ISO audit reports to independent peer reviewers[66]. At the same time, another COVID-19 'landmark' paper on the use of ACE-inhibitors and ARBS in COVID-19 was also retracted because the authors did not have access to raw data and data was not disclosed to auditors[32,67]. Although news in the media is often retracted, this came as a shock to the academic and medical communities who trust the tenets of evidence-based science, transparency, and authenticity[66,67,68,69,70]. However, it exposes an important reality. The chaos of the COVID-19 pandemic has affected the infrastructure of even the most trusted of sources.

Politics aside, the retraction of this study opened up the floodgates for other clinical trials that would otherwise have been received with criticism and pushback to make their presence known. Understanding clinical practice guidelines and conducting critical appraisal of the literature is *not* the responsibility of the educated citizen who should (under normal non-pandemic circumstances) trust evidence provided by reputable sources. However, this *is* a reminder to physicians and scientists to fairly adjudicate credibility regardless of institutional prestige and reputation. Here, the underlying theme of this manifesto is reverberated: the COVID-19 pandemic is the great equalizer, empowering for a few and humbling for many. As for HCQ, as more evidence mounts to build a case for its appropriate dose, target population, and outcome, it has promise in the current pandemic and future viral outbreaks, with or without the almighty 'Vaccine.'

VII. DECLASSIFIED INFORMATION
VACCINES & HOW CLINICAL TRIALS WORK

I know not with what weapons World War III will be fought, but World War IV will be fought with sticks and stones.

—Albert Einstein
Drafted the Russell-Einstein Manifesto Highlighting the Dangers of Nuclear Weapons During WWII. German Physicist of Jewish Ancestry Who Developed the Theory of Relativity & Mass-Energy Equivalence (World's Most Famous Equation, $E=mc^2$). Nobel Laureate for the Discovery of the Photoelectric Effect aka the Pivotal Step in Development of Quantum Theory…and, reportedly, *C Student*.

The development of a vaccine typically takes years to decades, case in point the Ebola vaccine. The first Ebola outbreak was in the 1970s, and an FDA-approved vaccine was not available until over 40 years later in 2019[71]. For some viruses like HIV, a vaccine has yet to be developed in spite of 30+ years of bleeding-heart advocacy and well-funded research efforts[72]. Even though the prospect of a SARS-CoV-2 vaccine is a central focus of COVID-19 media coverage, the jury is still out as to whether COVID-19 will safely *and* effectively fare any different from its predecessors.

Since we do not know what weapons we need to win every battle in COVID-19, we are throwing everything and the kitchen sink into ending the war. But, ending it may not be an option until there is a vaccine. If the audacity of social uproar for the expectation of immediate gratification topples critical thinking and perseverance, our next war may indeed be fought with sticks and stones.

HOW STUFF REALLY WORKS

Taking a vaccine from idea to fruition to clinical trial is an arduous process, hence why the average rate of vaccine development is just over 5%[73]. For those select few, there are inherent concerns. Will the vaccine be ineffective or worsen the disease? Who should be first to receive the vaccine, frontline healthcare workers or high-risk populations in the community? Will the success or failure of the vaccine in high-risk populations be similar in the general population? An important question also arises for vaccine developers. What is the safest, most effective way to design a clinical trial to fast track a vaccine to become available in months rather than years?

The concept of 'challenge trials' where volunteers receive a vaccine and are then challenged by receiving live virus may hasten results but has obvious ethical concerns[74]. Umbrella trials where multiple vaccines are tested in one clinical trial have been attempted in HIV, tuberculosis, and malaria but to no avail as a result of logistical hurdles[75]. With regards to clinical trials specifically designed for a COVID-19 vaccine, aside from efficacy and safety outcomes, exploratory outcomes of the trend in inflammatory and immune system biomarkers in cytokine storming are key as well. As far as traditional and experimental vaccine types go, RNA vaccines are cultivating interest[76]. RNA is implanted into a vector (microscopic vessel to deliver the therapeutic element) such as nano-sized lipid (fat) particles. When administered, the RNA message is 'translated' to DNA by the host cell and triggers the immune system to produce antibodies against the pathogen.

In addition to vaccines, moves are being made to create an 'antiserum'[77,78]. Yes, it is the tale of comic books and Hollywood biological warfare, I know. Antiserum is made by concentrating antibodies from convalescent plasma through specialized purification procedures that amplify potency. To increase yield, large animals like horses and cows are given this concentrate. After a period of time, usually weeks, the animal produces more serum. In the worst case scenario, sometimes the animal gets sick or dies. The highest risk has been in horses producing snake venom antiserum. Although pharmaceutical and biotechnology companies are in an arms race to develop an antiserum or antibody cocktail, clinical trials are months away and warranted ethical considerations for animal welfare will surely deter the enthusiasm of many.

Approved, Established Vaccines[79]

Type	Pros	Cons	Examples
Live-Attenuated	Weakened live version of pathogen creates long-lasting immunity. Usually 1-2 doses for lifetime immunity.	Contraindicated in people with weakened immune systems. Limited in countries without reliable refrigeration.	Yellow Fever Chickenpox Smallpox Rotavirus Measles Mumps Rubella
Inactivated	Better tolerated by people with weakened immune systems. More flexible storage requirements than live vaccines.	Killed version of pathogen does not confer long-term immunity. Need booster shots during lifetime.	Rabies Hepatitis A Flu Polio
Subunit, Recombinant, Polysaccharide, Conjugate	Key element of pathogen—protein, sugar, or capsid (encasing)—provides strong immunity. Well-tolerated by people with weakened immune systems and chronic disease.	Need booster shots over a lifetime for ongoing protection.	Hepatitis B Pneumococcal Meningococcal Shingles HPV Whooping Cough (Tdap) Haemophilus Influenza Type B
Toxoid	Toxin made by pathogen confers immunity by impairing part of virulent portion rather than the whole pathogen.	Booster shots needed over a lifetime for ongoing immunity.	Diphtheria Tetanus

Emerging, Experimental Vaccines

Type	Pros	Cons	Examples
DNA[80]	Produces strong, long-term immunity without risk of infection. Inexpensive and 'easy' to produce with reliable stability for storage. Replaces need for recombinant proteins and toxin agents.	Not commercially available in humans but clinical trials are ongoing. Risk to genes that affect human cell growth. Risk of stimulating antibody production against self-DNA.	West Nile Virus (Veterinary Vaccine Approved in Horses)
Recombinant Vector (Platform-Based)	Combines unrelated-pathogen with DNA of target pathogen and acts like real infection to train the immune system to fight.	Theoretically confers long-term immunity but too early to tell given novel nature.	Ebola Zaire, Approved 2019 On-going Human Trial[81]
RNA[82]	No genome integration because RNA 'translated' outside of the nucleus. Non-coding regions of RNA 'engineered' to increase translation. Easy to produce large quantities because *in vitro* production guarantees 'batch-to-batch' reproducibility.	Trigger for autoantibodies vis-à-vis an inflammatory response in people at risk, although less likely to trigger autoantibodies than DNA.	None approved for human use.
T-Cell Receptor Peptide[83,84]	Modulates cytokine production and cell-mediated immunity.	Unknown	Experimental models in valley fever, atopic dermatitis, MS

THE COVID-19 VACCINE: WHERE DO WE STAND?

A search in ClinicalTrials.gov results in 2,654 COVID-19 studies, which is just the tip of the iceberg (not including non-clinical trial research). Peer-reviewed journals are inundated with COVID-19 submissions, and papers are being expedited for publication. It is indeed the recipe for a perfect storm. According to the World Health Organization, over 100 vaccine candidates exist for COVID-19, most of which are just on paper[75]. Vaccine development takes years and a study drug almost always needs to complete the phase 3 clinical trial stage to be considered for FDA approval. Presently, there are 10 active, viable clinical trial candidates in the running to become the first COVID-19 vaccine.

Four inactivated vaccines are in phase 1 clinical trials using weakened or killed SARS-CoV-2. Two messenger RNA vaccines are in phase 2 clinical trials. One protein subunit vaccine is in the phase 1 clinical trial stage. The modus operandi of these candidates, as well as many other pre-clinical vaccines, is triggering an immune response from the infamous Spike protein, which as previously discussed, is the protein that aids and abets SARS-CoV-2 in binding to ACE and invading target host cells.

Two recombinant vaccines using primate adenovirus to carry DNA to Spike are underway as phase 2 and 2b/3 clinical trials. Although this is the most advanced phase of a COVID-19 vaccine trial, an adenovirus-based vaccine has never been approved in the US or Europe. Prior adenovirus vaccines were unsuccessful because people had pre-existing immunity to this common DNA adenovirus that causes run-of-the-mill problems such as pink eye, sore throat, diarrhea, and urinary tract infections. Regardless, the hope is that using the adenovirus approach will produce a strong immune system response of memory B cell and T cells. Given that the mechanism of a T-cell receptor peptide vaccine is modulation of cytokine production and cell-mediated immunity, this holds at least theoretical potential. There are no live-attenuated or toxoid vaccines in development.

So now, with a heightened appreciation for the time and elegance required for *successful* vaccine development, we will discuss current treatments and alternative medicines that hold both promise to buy us time and harbor limitations that set realistic expectations.

Clinical Trial Stage	Study Goals
Preclinical Research	To perform experimental, non-human research in a laboratory to understand the mechanism of action of a drug.
Phase 0	To learn how a drug works in the human body at a very low dose in a very small group of 10-15 people.
Phase I	To determine the optimal dosage of a drug given from low to high doses in a small group of 15-30 people.
Phase II	To validate safety and early efficacy in a larger group people with the disease or at risk for the disease *not* compared to current standard of care for the disease.
Phase III	To compare the effectiveness of a drug compared to standard of care as well as assess side effects in 100+ people. People may be assigned a treatment group (new drug versus standard of care) by random chance (randomization) to limit bias. **Usually needed before FDA approval[85].**
Phase IV	To test new drugs approved by the FDA in hundreds to thousands of people to determine short and long-term safety over time.

COVID-19 Vaccine Development[75]

Vaccine Type	Number of Trials	Trial Phase
RNA	2	1/2 and 2
Inactivated	4	1 and 1/2
Recombinant	2	2 and 2b/3
Protein Subunit	1	1/2
DNA	1	1

VIII. DRUG ARSENAL

PLASMA, TOCILIZUMAB, REMDESIVIR & CO.

I asked myself about the present: how wide it was, how deep it was, how much was mine to keep.

—Slaughterhouse-Five by Kurt Vonnegut
Mechanical Engineer & WWII Veteran Who Survived the Bombing of Dresden by Hiding in a Slaughterhouse Meat Locker

Resources in a pandemic are limited, and the ethics of war are complex. Ultimately, there is a disconnect between the human nature of an individual wanting the 'most' and the 'best' and the collective reality of *actually* getting it. The reality is that the 'best' treatment for COVID-19 is unknown and new diseases are best fought on all fronts, not just one. Although the media hypes up and misrepresents the 'latest' as also being the 'greatest,' they are *not* one in the same. Believe it or not, bread-and-butter supportive care is the cornerstone for survival in severe COVID-19. Feeling confident in this reality allows educated citizens, concerned for the worst-case-scenario playing out for themselves or their loved ones, to rest assured that if push comes to shove, they will receive the effective treatment they *need* rather than or in addition to the touted treatment they covet.

Do *not* be fooled. For the most part, even the 'latest' treatments are *not* new. Similar to most outbreaks, proposed 'cures' are simply old medicines studied for new indications, which is the case in remdesivir, tocilizumab, hydroxychloroquine, and convalescent plasma just to name a few. Rather, the development of new, disease-specific therapeutics (targeted antibodies, vaccines, antiserum, et cetera) occur concurrently and require lengthy and rigorous testing as well as extensive funding to assess safety and efficacy. Disease-specific treatments that make the cut may become widely used down the line if the target disease re-emerges *or* for another disease entirely. I hope you appreciate the irony here.

Such is the cycle of proposed cures, some of which have promise, many of which will come and go, and most of which have an M-O in parallel with the pathophysiology of many 'different' diseases. Treatments for COVID-19, similar to other viral diseases, are geared toward limiting viral replication at disease onset, mitigating severity of the body's inflammatory and immune response of the disease at its peak, and limiting the degree to which the immune system is weakened in the aftermath of disease and treatment.

STEROIDS

Steroids are low cost, easily accessible, and widely used medically (and recreationally). Steroids are made naturally in the body and play an essential role in development (progesterone), reproduction (testosterone, estrogen), growth and metabolism (cortisol), brain function (neurosteroids—DHEA), immunity (cholecalciferol), blood pressure and fluid control (mineralocorticoids), and the integrity of microscopic cell membranes (cholesterol). The principle concern in chronic steroid use is a decreased ability of the body to produce its own *endogenous* steroids and increased dependence on an outside, or *exogenous*, source with abrupt withdrawal triggering a 'crisis.' However, short-term use of steroids rarely causes dependence and, with regards to COVID-19, works effectively in mitigating the early and later signs of mild and severe COVID-19, respectively[86]. Moreover, concerns such as the development of diabetes and hypertension, weight gain, acne, and decreased bone density are relevant in chronic steroid use but negligible in the short-term in low-risk populations.

In pro-inflammatory conditions that activate the immune system, from infection to autoimmune diseases, the steroid family of choice is the glucocorticoids. Commonly used exogenous steroids with varying anti-inflammatory potencies and immunosuppressive profiles include prednisone taken by mouth, dexamethasone taken by mouth or IV, and methylprednisolone given IV. The use of steroids in infection may seem odd given its immunosuppressive properties. However, it is indeed standard of care in many life-threatening infections such as meningitis. In infectious diseases like COVID-19 that cause a fulminant inflammatory response known as the cytokine storm, high-dose, short-term IV glucocorticoids play an important adjunctive role in treatment[87,88]. As individual institutions continue to incorporate steroids into their COVID-19 treatment algorithm, clinical trials throughout the world, from China to the US, are under way to further investigate the role of steroids in COVID-19. For the treatment of mild COVID-19 in the hospital or community, the indication, population, dosing, and duration of treatment with steroids is not standardized.

REMDESIVIR

Remdesivir is designated by the FDA for the treatment of Ebola[89], has demonstrated efficacy against two other coronaviruses (MERS-CoV and SARS-CoV)[90], and was recently given emergency-use authorization by the FDA for use in COVID-19[91]. Remdesivir works by blocking RNA replication thereby limiting viral replication of many RNA viruses, including SAR-CoV-2, the virus that causes COVID-19. Remdesivir is currently used at many institutions. It is associated with kidney injury and will worsen existing kidney injury[92]. Most hospitals have different protocols for remdesivir administration based on whether a patient is intubated or not intubated, whereby they have a longer or shorter treatment course, respectively.

Recently published clinical trials[93] suggest effectiveness of remdesivir in treatment of COVID-19, but this is *not* without reservation. For example, one study showed that a 10-day course of remdesivir compared to placebo reduced recovery time in COVID-19. Unfortunately, patients did not have similar baseline characteristics. They had a range of presentations, from requiring little to no supplementary oxygen to having ventilator-dependent respiratory failure. And, of course, in patients with ventilator-dependent respiratory failure, the death rate was invariably high. This revisits a recurring theme that early evaluation, treatment, and delayed intubation trumps the promise of most treatments and interventions, regardless of their theoretical potential.

TOCILIZUMAB

Similar to other drugs that mitigate the cytokine storm in infectious diseases and inflammatory conditions, tocilizumab is an inhibitor of interleukin-6, or IL-6, which is markedly elevated in COVID-19[94,95]. As you know, IL-6 is a key pro-inflammatory cytokine that is measured and trended over time in hospitalized COVID-19 patients. Tocilizumab is FDA-approved for the treatment of autoimmune conditions including rheumatoid and juvenile arthritis and may be given to suppress IL-6 over-activity from T-cell therapies in leukemia and lymphoma[96]. High levels of IL-6 are also associated with other infectious diseases such as SARS, MERS, and influenza[97]. Recent COVID-19 studies suggest tocilizumab reduces IL-6 levels and improves some metrics of clinical outcome. For example, a recent study in China[98] demonstrated that tocilizumab was associated with a downward trend of several COVID-19 biomarkers including IL-6 and a clinical reduction in oxygen requirements. However, similar to remdesivir, these studies have several limitations, namely that very few patients were critically ill and intubated at treatment onset. By default, this cohort of patients will tend to do well regardless of specific treatments. Several clinical trials investigating tocilizumab are currently under way in countries with markedly different COVID-19 demographics, experiences, and outcomes, from Italy[99] to Switzerland[100]. And, in line with the COVID-19 cytokine storm 'chaser' movement, other cytokine inhibitor candidates such tumor necrosis factor-alpha (TNF-alpha) inhibitors presently used in inflammatory conditions such as rheumatoid arthritis, Crohn's disease, and psoriasis, are under investigation[101].

FAUX ACE

'Faux' ACE, scientifically known as rhACE-2, theoretically has strong potential at blocking SARS-CoV-2's first line of offense by binding to the *real* ACE receptor. As you know, the ACE receptor is the landing pad and entry point for SARS-CoV-2 to colonize and invade the body. RhACE-2 baits Spike (binding enhancement protein on SARS-CoV-2) and provides the virus with a false point of entry into its enemy target thereby mitigating invasion and neutralizing the enemy[102]. Pre-COVID-19, rhACE-2 was used for acute lung injury and shown to balance good versus bad ACE, decrease IL-6, and increase the anti-inflammatory and anti-microbial lung surfactant protein D (lung lubrication or 'soap')[103]. So far, experimental studies in COVID-19 using a hybrid protein made up of antibody fragments and rhACE-2 to neutralize SARS-CoV-2 suggest that rhACE-2 also confers cardiopulmonary protection in the heart and lungs. Clinical trials are underway[104,105].

PLASMA

And finally, la pièce de résistance: convalescent plasma for the treatment of COVID-19. Convalescent plasma has been used for over 100 years[106,107]. It is a form of passive immunity whereby previously infected people with antibodies transfer their antibodies to people who did not *actively* produce their own antibodies. Albeit temporary, the plasma is able to partially neutralize the pathogen. Plasma has shown benefit in hastening viral clearance in coronaviruses like MERS-CoV and SARS-CoV-2, as well as influenza, polio, measles, hepatitis B, Ebola, and, debatably, in rabies. Recent studies for its use in COVID-19 are positive but confounded by the concurrent use of other treatments like antivirals, antibiotics, and steroids. As is the case with any blood product, complications such as co-infection with another agent or adverse immune reactions resulting in hemodynamic instability or lung damage rarely occur[108].

Evidence suggests that ideal convalescent plasma candidates are early in their disease course, have less severe disease overall, or are at-risk without disease (frontline health care workers or direct caregivers of COVID-19 patients)[109]. In COVID-19 patients with more severe disease, there may be a paradoxical reaction whereby there is a secondary increase in viral load and dampening of the body's active immunity to the virus, making the use of convalescent plasma in these cases riskier, but still very worthwhile. And, from personal experience and early evidence in the COVID-19 ICU, critically ill patients have largely benefited from plasma. Numerous international and FDA-approved COVID-19 clinical trials are currently under way investigating the use of COVID-19 convalescent plasma in critical illness, non-critical illness, mild disease, prevention for at-risk people, and children[110,111,112]. This cumulative evidence will provide generalizable, reproducible, and valid evidence for or against the use of convalescent plasma on a larger scale.

Optimal timing of plasma administration and timeline of antibody development (IgG, IgM, or IgA) in COVID-19 are unclear. Standard requirements and site referrals may be found at American Association of Blood Banks[113], FDA COVID-19 Plasma Donation[114], and Mayo Clinic Expanded Access to Convalescent Plasma Program[115]. The Mayo Program and the FDA's Emergency Investigational New Drug (IND) proposal for convalescent plasma is now allowing physicians to provide patients with plasma as *part* of their COVID-19 treatment regimen. For plasma donation, requirements are as follows for potential donors[113,114,115]: documented SARS-CoV-2 infection, symptom-free status for 14 days, presence of antibodies at a sufficient level to confer immunity about 2 to 3 weeks following infection, and compliance with blood donation standards. A single donor can treat 2 to 3 recipients through a process of plasma extraction called plasmapheresis. As discussed in earlier, quantitative antibody tests are not widely available to ensure donors have sufficient level of antibodies rather than just positive/negative. And so, physicians and scientists must sometimes use clinical judgement in lieu of well-designed, flawlessly executed testing.

IX. ALCHEMY NOW

MELATONIN, VITAMIN D & ZINC + C

Water: 35 liters, carbon: 20 kilograms, ammonia: 4 liters, lime: 1.5 kilograms, phosphorus: 800 grams, salt: 250 grams, saltpeter: 100 grams, sulfur: 80 grams, fluorine: 7.5 grams, iron: 5.6 grams, silicon: 3 grams, and 15 other elements in small quantities. That is the total chemical makeup of the average adult body. Modern science knows all of this, but there has never been a single example of successful human transmutation. It's like there's some missing ingredient. Scientists have been trying to find it for hundreds of years, pouring tons of money into research, and to this day they don't have a theory. For that matter, the elements found in a human being are all junk that you can buy in any market with a child's allowance. Humans are pretty cheaply made.

—Fullmetal Alchemist, Vol. 1 by Hiromu Arakawa
   Japanese Manga Artist Influenced by the European Industrial Revolution and Social Paradigms of War, Family, Fellowship, Progress & Political Corruption

For the anthropocentric mind, it is humbling to think of yourself as an elixir of basic elements greater than the sum of your parts. On the other hand, an extraordinary sense of interconnectedness with everything comes from the acknowledgement that the 'star-stuff' that makes up each and every person and makes *us* 'us' was created long before and will exist even after nature takes it course. That being said, it is no wonder that so many elements in nature untouched by the human hand have the power to cure, agency to ignore, and means to kill us. And so, let us discuss some elements that are on our side against COVID-19.

MELATONIN

First and foremost, as any insomniac will tell you, melatonin is NOT a sleeping pill. Similar to the misrepresentation of hydroxychloroquine, general understanding of the *real* melatonin has been obscured by mismarketing. In fact, one of the initial motivations in writing this manifesto stems from the misconception of melatonin use in COVID-19 ICU patients in other frontline healthcare workers. During a causal conversation at 0300 in the COVID-19 ICU, two (rock star) nurses asked me why most intubated, heavily sedated COVID-19 patients had melatonin on their medication list. Earlier that day, one of the nurses asked a doctor 'why melatonin' and was given a 'because I told you so' type answer. Realizing no one really seemed to know why and wanting to do what was right for her patients, she started holding melatonin under the presumption it was prescribed in error. Being passionate about melatonin long before COVID-19, I jumped at the opportunity to right a wrong. Although it theoretically improves sleep quality and architecture of sedated, ICU patients and may decrease the need for heavy sedation, this was *not* why COVID-19 ICU patients were on melatonin.

Melatonin is a hormone made naturally in the brain's pineal gland, anecdotally known as the 'third eye,' and other important parts of the brain. Melatonin regulates our 24-hour circadian rhythm, or biological clock, as well as 'CLOCK' genes essential in epigenetics, aging, disease, longevity, and healthspan[116]. In addition to CLOCK genes, melatonin is involved in other longevity pathways, and, for our purposes...drum roll...preventing injury to the lungs from an infectious agent. This latter function is not as far-removed as it seems from the principal roles of melatonin. The anti-infective properties of melatonin are, in fact, a result of its omnipotent cytokine storm-chasing abilities[117].

Numerous randomized controlled trials have shown that melatonin in a variety of doses and different lengths of treatment decreases key inflammatory markers including interleukin-6 (IL-6), IL-1 beta, tumor necrosis factor-alpha (TNF-α), high sensitivity C-reactive protein (hsCRP), and lipoperoxidase in people with a wide range of inflammatory conditions including multiple sclerosis[118], diabetes mellitus[119], physical stressors of surgery[120], acute heart attack[121], and periodontitis[122]. The reason melatonin is able to regulate a diverse range of inflammatory biomarkers is the result of its opportune position in an upstream anti-inflammatory pathway: sirtuin-1, or SIRT-1. In addition to being a prime regulator of cell longevity and lifespan[123], SIRT-1 works with other proteins and gatekeepers such as toll-like receptor 4 or—TLR4 and the survivor activating factor enhancement pathway[124] to mitigate inflammation.

In a cytokine storm from an infectious disease such as COVID-19, this pathway confers protection against septic shock and sepsis-induced lung, kidney, heart, and liver injury. With a stronghold in so many aspects of the cytokine storm, melatonin is a formidable opponent of the 'inflammasome'[125] during peak inflammation and has been studied in lung diseases including influenza A virus[126], syncytial virus[127], bacterial toxin-induced lung injury[128], allergic airway inflammation[129], and oxygen-induced lung injury from over-ventilation[130]. From a neurological perspective during a cytokine storm, melatonin confers protection by reducing the brain's inflammatory response and fortifying the brain-blood barrier to prevent pathogen invasion[131].

In addition to inflammation, melatonin also limits excess growth factor release into the circulation to prevent fibrosis (thickening) and stenosis (narrowing) of blood vessels in the heart, brain, and other vital organs. Melatonin fights oxidative stress via activating the potent antioxidant superoxide dismutase, deactivating the pro-oxidant nitric oxide synthase, and serving as a free radical scavenger. In the immune system, melatonin enhances the immune response and fosters the growth and development of natural killer cells (yes, that's a thing).

Regarding safety, pre-COVID-19 clinical trials in ICU patients and healthy people show that even at high doses melatonin is very well-tolerated[132]. Any stipulation is *not* with safety, but rather, the potential that high dose supplementation desensitizes the brain's ability to produce its own melatonin independently, thereby becoming dependent on exogenous melatonin. However, this is only relevant in healthy people taking daily melatonin. In critical illness, the gravity of the situation warrants a 'bet-the-farm' approach. In light of the aforementioned benefits of melatonin, it is no wonder that clinical trials investigating it as a treatment for COVID-19[133] as well as prophylaxis against COVID-19 in healthy people[134] and frontline healthcare workers are underway.

VITAMIN D

Cholecalciferol, known as the active form of vitamin D, is a steroid hormone that plays an essential role in the immune system and is a staple element in the regimen of many people with autoimmune diseases such as multiple sclerosis. Vitamin D also has several targeted roles in modulating the immune system in infectious diseases such as COVID-19. Vitamin D mitigates the inflammatory response in COVID-19 by competing with SARS-CoV-2 for ACE receptors, which as you know is the landing pad and entry point for SARS-CoV-2 to invade the body[135]. The relationship between vitamin D and ACE is well-known and studied in the autoimmune, pro-inflammatory disease sarcoidosis. In the respiratory tract, vitamin D also enhances the ability of epithelial cells ('skin' or epithelium of the lungs) to produce antimicrobial proteins that further mitigate infection[136].

Vitamin D levels are notoriously low in the general population, with certain populations like dark-skinned people affected to a greater degree given a decreased ability to absorb precursors to active vitamin D from the sun. With most people staying indoors more than accustomed, whether from quarantine or working remotely, deficiencies may become more clinically significant. In fact, government agencies in countries such as the UK recommend vitamin D supplementation during seasons where people would normally have more sun exposure[137]. In this case, it is worth stating that more is *not* better. High doses of vitamin D supplementation should be reserved for people with medical conditions warranting high-dose supplementation under the supervision of a physician. Fat-soluble vitamins such as vitamins A, D, and E have the rare potential to reach toxic levels in the body when taken at (absurdly) high doses. This is in contrast to water-soluble vitamins such as B complex and vitamin C that with some exception (beware of B6) do not reach toxic levels. But certainly, eating vitamin D-rich foods and *modest* supplementation are reasonable not only in the COVID-19 era but for general immune system health and well-being. Evidence in the literature for the role vitamin D in infectious disease pre-COVID-19 is generally positive. A critical appraisal of a series of high quality clinical trials demonstrated that vitamin D confers protection against acquiring respiratory infections in people with very low vitamin D levels (<25 nmol/L)[138]. As a testament to the importance of risk factor management in disease prevention, a large study cleverly entitled COVIDENCE UK is currently investigating how diet and lifestyle, including vitamin D status, effect SARS-CoV-2 transmission, severity, recovery, and long term effects[139].

ZINC & VITAMIN C

Zinc is a trace element essential for survival. It plays an integral role in over 3000 functions in the body including DNA and RNA metabolism, cell communication, gene expression, and programmed cell death. Zinc homeostasis occurs in the gut, and zinc is found in the eyes, brain, muscle, bones, kidney, liver, and, in very high concentrations, the semen. When zinc homeostasis is disrupted, bad things happen. For example, when in-sync, zinc enhances neuroplasticity, and when out-of-sync, zinc leads to neurotoxicity. In infectious diseases such as COVID-19, zinc has a preventive and adjunctive treatment role via its properties of immunomodulation, anti-inflammation, limiting ventilator-induced lung injury, and improving mucous clearance[140,141].

Cells have natural transporters called zip proteins that help zinc enter cells to kill the virus. In fact, as discussed earlier, hydroxychloroquine (HCQ) is a 'zinc ionophore[142].' This means that HCQ is a synthetic doorway that allows more zinc to enter cells and kill more virus. Not surprisingly, zinc decreases the activity of ACE, the receptor for SARS-CoV-2, thereby augmenting the body's ability to prevent infection. If the virus breaches these lines of security and invades, the next line of defense is mitigating the cytokine storm. Zinc increases anti-inflammatory cytokines, decreases pro-inflammatory cytokines, and reroutes rogue pathways. Zinc also reduces the risk of a concurrent bacterial infection in the lungs. By fortifying the respiratory epithelial barrier, zinc improves the clearance of mucous from cilia, or hair-like projections, in the respiratory tract. This proposed anti-bacterial effect is demonstrated in common bacterial infections such as streptococcal pneumonia. High-risk groups known to be zinc deficient include people who are obese, diabetic, or have coronary artery disease. Studies are presently ongoing to further investigate the promising role of zinc in COVID-19, both as monotherapy and combined with other elements, namely vitamin C[143,144].

Vitamin C is best known for its antioxidant properties and role as a scavenger of rogue pro-oxidants in inflammatory processes from infection to immune dysfunction, hence its presence in most over-the-counter cold remedies. During infection, vitamin C levels become depleted and requirements increase with increasing severity of infection. Studies long before COVID-19 investigating high-dose IV vitamin C have yielded mixed results[145], and studies investigating high-dose IV vitamin C for COVID-19 are ongoing in countries such as China[146]. Given its lack of specificity to the mechanism of action of COVID-19, vitamin C supplementation is safe, but it is not a standalone deterrent of COVID-19. It best serves a sidekick role next to elements such a vitamin D, zinc, melatonin, et cetera.

The reality is, however, that in spite of pre-COVID-19 widespread commercial availability, good safety profiles, and evidence-based efficacy, many hospitals and drug stores ran out of these adjunctive treatments very early on in the pandemic. Albeit unsettling, in the severely ill the rat race reaches far beyond the rationing of alternative medicines. It courses into the realm of stone-cold survival needs vis-à-vis the ventilator.

X. THE GREAT DICTATOR

VENTILATORS, PRONING, ARDS, HPV & HAPE!#%&$?

Soldiers! Don't give yourselves to brutes, men who despise you, enslave you, who regiment your lives, tell you what to do, what to think, and what to feel! Who drill you, diet you, treat you like cattle, use you as cannon fodder. Don't give yourselves to these unnatural men—machine men with machine minds and machine hearts! You are not machines! You are not cattle! You are men!

—The Final Speech by Charlie Chaplin
   Father of Silent Film, Star of the Great Dictator, Survivor of Familial Warfare & Poverty

In a pandemic, one of the many purposes flattening the curve serves is to gauge how an unmitigated surge in cases strains the chain of supply and demand. In COVID-19, ventilator supply and ICU bed availability is *the* rate-limiting step. Globally, ventilators dictate how systems of care, from a community hospital in a developing country to an academic institution in New York City, handle their most severe cases of COVID-19. In some cases, objective measures (age, pre-existing conditions, et cetera) and subjective measures (a person's 'value' to society, number of dependents, et cetera) impact who gets what, whether intentionally or subconsciously. Needless to say, the ethical implications here are far-reaching as man's real-time dependence on machine comes to a climax before our eyes.

This is where mitigation strategies are instrumental. Flattening the curve by delaying and suppressing the peak results in the same number of cases but over a more stable time course, thereby reducing peak demand for ventilators and providing time for increased ventilator production. In a more cooperative world and country, a centralized ventilator inter-state 'transfer system' is one of many possible solutions to address need during asynchronous peaks in different regions in space and time. In the US, governmental agencies have not yet opted to engage in increased ventilator production, although some industries such are shifting production to ventilators through the Defense Production Act. This law was enacted decades ago at the start of the Korean War and has been reauthorized dozens of times during periods of crisis, from the Cold War to COVID-19.

THE VENTILATOR

Pneumonia in COVID-19 is a red herring[147]. COVID-19 causes low oxygen levels throughout the body, but, by nature of the beast, presents most dramatically in the lungs. In people who decompensate from pneumonia to respiratory failure, autopsy of the lungs reveals inflammation, damage, and fluid in alveoli (millions of tiny sacs in the lungs that exchange air) surrounded by hyaline membranes (proteins and dead cells lining alveoli). This is pathognomonic for the well-known syndrome that continues to make headlines during the COVID-19 pandemic: acute respiratory distress syndrome, or ARDS. From case reports of successful lung transplants[148] to leaks of unprecedented findings[149], the truth is, COVID-19 is *not* your typical ARDS. As such, for both the physician and educated citizen, the importance of understanding the art and science of ventilator management in COVID-19 is beyond compare.

As an erratically beeping, cryptic box with foreign acronyms and livestreaming graphs attached to a comatose person, a ventilator is intimidating. So, let us break down the box. First off, most COVID-19 patients in the hospital do *not* need to be on the ventilator[150]. The rate of intubation is less than 10%, and the goal is to *delay* intubation for as long as safely possible. Up to 90% of patients on the ventilator are unable to be successfully extubated and/or avoid tracheostomy placement. A unique subset of COVID-19 patients 'electively' intubated for a procedure or surgery directly or indirectly related to a complication of COVID-19 usually do *not* have a severe respiratory-predominant form of COVID-19 and are extubated easier than their sicker counterparts.

Ventilator settings, or modes, have classically been divided into those that control lung volume or lung pressure. However, modern ventilator modes combine characteristics of both volume and pressure control. In COVID-19, the goals are to optimize the 'trigger' for a breath, limit the size of a breath, and time the duration of a breath. This limits work of breathing, synchronizes breathing with the ventilator, and lowers the peak lung pressure. This streamlines the work of the heart and maximizes blood flow to other organs. Optimizing a measure termed 'PEEP' is also important to recruit alveoli in lung injury. If PEEP is too low, alveoli are not recruited, heart output is poor, and blood flow to other organs is diminished. If PEEP is too high, alveoli are over-recruited, barotrauma ensues, and there is damage to healthy lung tissue. On the whole, combined lung-protective ventilation strategies are intended to not over-oxygenate, not over-inflate, and not over-work the lungs and body as a whole.

Methods to Delay Intubation

Severity	Non-Invasive Ventilation	Mechanisms of Action
Mild	Room Air (RA)	Observation of patient breathing naturally on RA.
	Nasal Cannula (NC)	Oxygen measured in liters is delivered through nostril prongs to maintain oxygen levels at a goal which varies from greater than 86% to 96%.
Moderate	High Flow Oxygen (HFO) & Non-Rebreather (NR) Mask	When patients do not meet O2 goal with NC, the HFO or NR mask is placed to provide higher concentration of oxygen to meet goal.
High	Continuous Positive Airway Pressure (CPAP)	Continuous pressurized air is delivered through a physically obstructed airway in patients able to breathe spontaneously and independently. Pro: Recruits more lung surface area by opening alveoli for ventilation, similar to PEEP. Con: Because of a uniform pressure, may be difficult to exhale against.
	Bi-Level Positive Airway Pressure (BiPAP)	Dual pressures for inspiration and exhalation allow more air to go in and out of the lungs. Pro: May be more useful than CPAP in low oxygen levels, heart and lung dysfunction, and nerve-muscle disease. Con: Risk of aspiration in the poorly responsive patient or patient unable to manage secretions given a breath may be delivered by BiPAP independent of spontaneous breathing.

Goals of Ventilator Management

Stage	Process	Mechanism
Intubation	Pressure-Control, Volume-Control, and Hybrids Modes	Common modes in COVID-19 are 'PRVC' and 'APRV' with heavy sedation to facilitate synchrony with the ventilator, decreased work of breathing, and optimization of alveolar recruitment. Settings based on metrics such as ideal body weight and pH of the lungs and body.
Weaning	'CPAP' and 'Pressure Support' trials while intubated.	Weaning from dependent modes of breathing to modes requiring patient to initiate spontaneous breathing on an ongoing, trial basis.
Extubation	Breathing tube and ventilator are successfully removed.	A process requiring patient alertness, ability to protect airway, ability to self-oxygenate and ventilate as well as supporting objective data from chest x-ray and ABG.
Tracheostomy	Breathing tube and ventilator cannot safely be removed and/or complications of prolonged intubation are present.	Reversible in patients with good to guarded prognosis at which time patient can be 'decannulated' or have tracheostomy tube removed. In COVID-19, many hospital protocols mandate negative repeat COVID-19 testing prior to tracheostomy.

THE PRONING POSITION

Proning involves repositioning a person from the supine (belly up) to prone (belly down) position. Many patients with mild COVID-19 self-prone, whereas in critically ill patients who are paralyzed and sedated, there is a trained team devoted to proning and supining patients efficiently and safely. Proning is shown to be more effective in COVID-19 pneumonia than traditional ARDS. Because blood flow to the lungs is impaired in COVID-19 pneumonia, proning allows more lung regions to perfuse and ventilate. Although early intubation is key in dire straits, in more stable people teetering on the edge, delaying extubation is ideal. Proning often provides the opportunity to delay intubation. Recent studies show that in non-intubated people, oxygen levels improve after just a few minutes of self-proning, with the main limitation being physical intolerance of the proned position[151,152]. In intubated patients, correct patient selection, timing, and duration of proning are all important variables. For now, evidence suggests that in patients with low oxygen levels for an extended period of time, initiation of proning very soon after intubation for a duration of at least 12 hours is optimal[153].

ACUTE RESPIRATORY DISTRESS SYNDROME

Features that distinguish COVID-19 from ARDS are relatively mild respiratory symptoms compared to a severe constellation of signs including: profoundly low oxygen levels in the blood; very abnormal imaging of the lungs; very high oxygen requirements; and preserved lung compliance (lungs' ability to stretch and expand). There is also more pulmonary shunting where poorly oxygenated blood in fluid-overloaded alveoli circulates between the lungs perpetuating a vicious cycle of oxygen deprivation[154].

HYPOXIC PULMONARY VASOCONSTRICTION

In severe COVID-19, the degree of hypoxia (low oxygen in the lungs and body) and hypoxemia (low oxygen in the blood) are out of proportion to actual lung injury[155,156]. This points to an underlying problem in the body's 'homeostatic oxygen-sensing system,' or HOSS. The HOSS system includes parts of the lungs, carotid arteries, adrenal glands, and 'brain' cells outside of the brain. When the lungs are deprived of oxygen in a disease such as severe pneumonia, their normal reaction is to restrict blood flow in injured lung tissue to preserve blood flow to salvageable lung tissue. This concept is known as hypoxic pulmonary vasoconstriction, or HPV[157].

HPV optimizes ventilation-to-perfusion (oxygenation-to-blood flow). The carotids have mitochondria-powered sensors that detect low oxygen levels and increase our instinctive drive to breathe. Interestingly, many proteins involved in COVID-19 are associated with mitochondria, otherwise known as the cell's oxygen powerhouse or energy factory. This strengthens the case for the presence of hypoxemia out of proportion to lung injury in severe COVID-19. In COVID-19, the protective HPV response is blunted by factors such as the high inflammatory states that dilate blood vessels thereby not allowing for life-saving blood rationing, increased dead space in the lungs, and micro-clots (remember the pro-clotting state in COVID-19).

HIGH ALTITUDE PULMONARY EDEMA

In high altitude pulmonary edema (HAPE), blood vessel constriction is exaggerated and disorganized[158]. Constriction of the veins, not arteries, in the lungs is a distinguishing factor from HPV. Constricted veins cause back flow, increase lung pressure, and perpetuate alveolar leakage. This is in contrast to HPV, where lung pressures are low and arteries are constricted in damaged areas and dilated in salvageable areas. HAPE is primarily a blood flow problem causing high pressures and edema. This is in contrast to ARDS associated with high lung pressures and edema secondary to a pro-clotting, pro-inflammatory state.

Although COVID-19 shares characteristics of ARDS, HPV, and HAPE, much controversy surrounds equating the three[159]. The truth is, patients with severe COVID-19 pneumonia likely experience each of these disease processes on a spectrum during their disease course, and it is imperative for the frontline doctor to be able to distinguish between these distinct entities in order to modify and optimize treatment over time. For example, treating HAPE with a blood vessel dilator may be harmful in HPV. Similarly, treating HPV with carotid body activators (almitrine) or medications that prevent over-dilation (indomethacin, nitric oxide inhibitors, methyl arginine analogs) may be harmful in HAPE or ARDS. Although difficult to implement due to contamination issues, bedside testing with ultrasound of the heart and lung blood vessels may serve as an objective way to distinguish between ARDS, HPV, and HAPE as well as guide treatment of other organs affected by COVID-19, which we will now review.

XI. ORGAN STRIKE

KIDNEY PUNCH, GUTS & THE MEDULLA OBLONGATA

Battles are won by slaughter and maneuver. The greater the general, the more he contributes in maneuver, the less he demands in slaughter.

—Winston S. Churchill
Brought Renown to the Concept of the *Iron Curtain*, Prime Minister of the UK, WWII Army Officer, Experience in the Anglo-Indian War, Anglo-Sudan War, Second Boer War & WWI, Economic Liberal, Imperialist, Champion of Prison Reform & Workers' Social Security

A COVID-19 organ strike, akin to a military strike, is a soldiered operation other than war intended to deter war and promote peace with more restrictive rules of engagement[160]. The body is cognizant enough to gauge when continued combat against an infectious agent will result in irreversible damage from multiorgan failure. As such, organs may opt to stop fighting and engage in more productive exchanges. Unfortunately, in the case of COVID-19, the reality is we are *not* there yet. We are still very much in the war and first need to have a fundamental understanding of what COVID-19 can do to the body before we solider on for peace.

KIDNEY PUNCH

The kidneys are responsible for filtering out toxins and excess fluid from the body. Kidney failure is not compatible with life unless it is reversible or amendable to dialysis. Dialysis involves a machine working as an artificial kidney outside the body to filter blood and return it back to the body. People on dialysis prior to COVID-19 infection are at higher risk for a more severe disease course for several reasons, from exposure to other immunocompromised people at dialysis centers to chronically damaged blood vessels susceptible to cytokine storming. Also, because COVID-19 preferentially attacks the kidneys and many potential treatments for severe COVID-19 and non-COVID-19 related ICU complications are contraindicated in severe kidney disease, these people are at a significant disadvantage[161]. In mild cases of COVID-19, protein loss in the urine occurs in nearly half of cases at the time of ER evaluation. This is a conservative estimate because baseline kidney function is often unknown. For people who develop severe COVID-19 and fluid overload refractory to conservative management, nearly half progress to significant kidney injury and approximately one-fourth of those people need dialysis two weeks into their hospital course[162]. Gentle forms of dialysis where fluid is removed slowly is preferred to avoid hemodynamic instability. As in chronic dialysis, the need for urgent dialysis in and of itself a poor marker of survival. Very importantly, dialysis does *not* affect antibody treatments because antibody size exceeds the size of elements that can be removed in dialysis[162].

The Current Understanding of How Kidney Injury Works in Severe COVID-19[162]

Source of Injury	Mechanisms
Heart Failure	Severe heart injury, by means of direct toxicity from the virus or cytokine storm, sequelae of lung injury, or hemodynamic instability, invariably occurs in severe COVID-19. The risk is multiplied in people with underlying heart conditions. The kidneys share a co-dependent relationship with the heart, and heart injury leads to pump failure and back flow leads to kidney congestion and damage.
Volume Loss	Severe dehydration results from 'third-spacing.' Third-spacing occurs when protein and fluid are exiled from blood vessels to soft tissue resulting in volume depletion and malnourishment, often with a misleadingly 'bloated' volume-overloaded appearance. Also, dehydration from 'insensible losses' in fever lead to poor blood flow, oxygen, and nutrient delivery to kidneys resulting in injury.
ACE and Viral Invasion	ACE is highly concentrated in the kidneys where it serves as the SARS-CoV-2 receptor in the lining of kidney 'tubing.' ACE and the virus cause cells in the tube lining to die and become necrotic. This tubular necrosis leaves sediment in the urine and is one of the main reasons patients go into acute kidney failure requiring dialysis.
Podocyte Damage	Amoeba-like cells that protect the kidney-blood barrier (similar to the blood-brain barrier) called podocytes are directly damaged by SARS-CoV-2 resulting in a mass exodus of protein from the body that is then wasted in the urine, known as proteinuria.
Hypercoagulability	A pro-clotting, or hypercoagulable state, and low oxygen levels lead to micro-clots and micro-strokes in the kidneys, respectively.
Nephrotoxicity	Avoidance of medications that are nephrotoxic, or toxic to the kidneys, is important. Many antibiotics and vasopressors (IV continuous infusions used in critically ill patients to maintain blood pressure high enough to perfuse the body) can be nephrotoxic. They may be substituted for less nephrotoxic agents in a similar class.
Metabolic Acidosis	Diligently replacing fluid losses with just the right amount of electrolytes and protein, mainly albumin, and correcting low pH in the blood, known as metabolic acidosis, are protective to the heart and kidneys.

FOMITE-O-PHOBIA? NO GUTS, NO GLORY

A subset of people develops gastrointestinal symptoms from COVID-19, including diarrhea, nausea, vomiting, and less commonly liver injury. Studies have shown SARS-CoV-2 can be detected from mouth to anus, after somehow surviving the acidic environment of the stomach. The virus can often be detected in the feces of a COVID-19 positive person with or without gastrointestinal symptoms, and there is often prolonged fecal shedding whereby fecal samples remain positive after respiratory samples are negative[27]. So, why and how?

Remember, ACE is the receptor for SARS-CoV-2. ACE happens to be an important regulator of intestinal inflammation and is highly produced in the gastrointestinal tract. Interestingly, studies have shown that successful viral entry is not just dependent on ACE but also an enzyme that activates the Spike protein of coronaviruses, which is also highly produced in the gastrointestinal tract. As such, people with inflammatory diseases of the bowel may be at increased risk of a more severe gastrointestinal course. On the other hand, people without previous gastrointestinal disease who have a gastrointestinal-predominant form of COVID-19 typically have a more benign course

Early and adequate nutrition is also paramount in mitigating COVID-19, namely preventing protein loss. In the hospital, nutritional status is assessed by albumin blood levels and protein levels in the urine[163]. As we just learned, third-spacing secondary to protein loss in the urine and protein extravasation out of the blood vessels and into the soft tissue, is the emblem of poor nutritional status. In critically ill, intubated COVID-19 patients, aggressive tube feeding with protein supplementation is often limited by intolerance and delayed gut motility. In these cases, TPN (IV food supplementation) is the next step with its own set of complications.

Similar to kidney disease, severe COVID-19 is also associated with liver dysfunction in previously healthy livers[164]. As such, people with chronic liver disease are at higher risk for a variety of reasons. The liver is responsible for producing albumin, clotting factors, insulin, and metabolizing a large number of medications. Low albumin, poor nutritional status, imbalanced pro- and anti-clotting factors, and under- or over-clearance of medications sets these people up for a more severe course of COVID-19. The liver is also adversely effected by many potential treatments for COVID-19, which are hepatotoxic, or toxic to the liver.

THE MEDULLA OBLONGATA

When the mind is dazed and confused, brain damaged, and nerves shot, the fortitude required to fight a disease that can wreak havoc on the body is multiplied 10-fold, hence the importance of mapping out what we know, what we do not know, and what we need to learn about how viral diseases such as COVID-19 affect the brain and nervous system. The most important concept is to understand that innumerable infections, from the flu to herpes, have the potential to cause a neurological disease, albeit rare in all instances. In the case of viral diseases like COVID-19, the *now* is complicated. As evidence is mounting for COVID-19, the development of clinical trials to investigate its neurological manifestations is lagging behind. With the exception of studies investigating the association of stroke and COVID-19[165], so far, the majority of evidence for other neurological diseases in COVID-19 is in the form of anecdotal case reports and observational studies. This has prompted brain specialists from all over the world to construct an international neuro-COVID-19 data registry, which will build epidemiological and mechanistic evidence needed to move forward[166]. Thankfully, much insight can be gained in understanding similar viruses with a comparable M-O. Scientists have found other coronaviruses, including MERS-CoV and SARS-CoV in the brains, particularly in the brainstem, of infected people and animals[167]. As you know, SARS-CoV-2 is genetically similar and seems to follow a similar pattern. A handful of institutions have even reported the presence of SARS-CoV-2 in the spinal fluid of living patients with COVID-19 who had negative nasal/oral testing[168,169].

The mechanism by which coronaviruses spread from the lungs to the brain is via a synapse-connected route to the breathing center of the brain: the medulla oblongata[170,171]. This mechanism is thought to be causative or significantly associated with the respiratory decline of some COVID-19 patients. This synapse-connected route is similar to West Nile virus[172], herpes[173], and swine flu that serves as a conduit to the central nervous system—brain and spinal cord; peripheral nervous system—nerves in the face, trunk, arms, and legs; and autonomic nervous system—carotid baroreceptors and sympathetic (fight) versus parasympathetic (flight) responses. Hence, it is an evolutionary goldmine for viral neurological invasion.

Breakdown of COVID-19 Disease State and Type of Neurological Disease[174]

Infectious State	Neurological Disease
Pro-Clotting State or Hypercoagulability	Ischemic Stroke: Blood clots block blood flow in brain arteries. Venous Thrombosis: Blood clots block blood flow in brain veins.
Anti-Clotting State or Thrombocytopenia/DIC	Brain Hemorrhage: Low platelets or dysfunctional blood coagulation cause spontaneous or provoked bleeding. `
Cytokine Storm	Coma: Inflammatory cascade and unmitigated oxidative stress 'shut down' the cortex. Brainstem disease: Inflammatory cascade and oxidative stress damage the brainstem. Necrotizing hemorrhagic encephalitis: Inflammatory cascade and oxidative stress directly destroy friable brain tissue from the outside-in leading to brain cell necrosis and bleeding. Seizure: Inflammatory cascade and oxidative stress lower the seizure threshold by increasing excitability and destabilizing brain cells. Spinal cord myelitis: Inflammatory cascade and oxidative stress cause inflammation and damage of the spinal cord. Encephalopathy/delirium: Inflammatory cascade and oxidative stress are toxic to brain cell function and communication leading to confusion and fluctuating levels of consciousness, especially with baseline poor 'neurological reserves.' Ataxia: Inflammatory cascade and oxidative stress damage high energy-requiring cells in the cerebellum. Headache, fatigue, generalized weakness, and malaise: Inflammatory cascade and oxidative stress uses up the brain and body's energy and increases the demand for more energy.
Peri- or Post-Viral Autoimmune Reactions	Coma: Self-antibodies attack the whole brain or parts of the brain that control wakefulness and arousal.

	Brainstem/limbic system disease: Self-antibodies attack the brainstem and lead to disinhibition, cranial nerve damage, or coma. Seizure: Self-antibodies trigger over-excitability and destabilization of brain cells. Guillain-Barre syndrome: Self-antibodies invade peripheral nerves and cause weakness in a 'stocking and glove' pattern. Encephalopathy/encephalitis: Self-antibodies invade brain fluid and infect the brain from the outside-in causing a range of symptoms from confusion to coma and death. Spinal cord myelitis: Self-antibodies attack the spinal cord and fluid leading to a range of signs and symptoms from pain to paralysis. Ataxia: Self-antibodies attack the cerebellum leading to imbalance and poor coordination.
Recrudescence of Chronic Neurological Problems[175]	Old viral infections: A weakened immune system indirectly reactivates 'inactive' or dormant viruses such as oral herpes, genital herpes, or trigeminal neuralgia. Old stroke symptoms: Poor neurological reserve allows infection to exacerbate minor deficits that were previously more severe (like running a marathon exacerbates chronic arthritis).

Now, *breathe*. In the grand scheme of things, the 'organ strike' is very rare. Aside from traditional risk factors such as high exposure and immunocompromise, however, COVID-19 does hold a few wild cards that again remind us to expect the unexpected.

XII. CASUALTIES OF WAR

TESTOSTERONE, YOUTH, KAWASAKI & COVID TOES

Truth, it has been said, is the first casualty of war.

—E.D. Morel
Leader of the WWI Pacifist Movement & Founder of the Congo Reform Association

Some things are far from the truth and solely by-products of society. Consequently, when aberrancies of nature like COVID-19 with no regard for stereotypes and tall tales of strong men, invincible children, and 'what doesn't kill you' strike, they tear the fabric of our cultural beliefs. The truth is, some men are weak, some children die, and some harsh realities are harder to accept the closer they are to home. The strategy here is to *not* feel defeated but, rather, to empower yourself with knowledge and bite the bullet of sad truths and hard facts.

THE TESTOSTERONE THEORY

In the microcosm of my personal experience, critically ill COVID-19 ICU patients were predominantly male. As opposed to being an anomaly, these findings are real and have prompted the development of scientific hypotheses and investigation of potential treatments. But first, here are some rough estimates. In the SARS-CoV-2 positive population, prevalence is slightly higher in males at just under 60%. In contrast, mortality from COVID-19 is significantly higher in males. When broken down by age bracket: over 80% of deaths in ages 30 to 39 are male; over 70% of deaths in ages 40 to 49 are male; nearly 80% of deaths in ages 50 to 79 are male; and almost 70% of deaths in ages 80 to 89 are male. There is mixed evidence as to why, but the malefactor seems to be the complex role of testosterone[176].

Unhealthy aging and diseases such as obesity, diabetes, coronary artery disease, sleep apnea, and COPD reduce testosterone. Normal testosterone levels are associated with increased lung capacity and improved peak oxygen consumption, which correlate with the vitality and virility we typically associate with testosterone. As we have learned, the SARS-CoV-2 receptor, ACE, is heavily concentrated in the lungs as well as male testosterone-producing cells in the testicles. But, this is only the beginning of the complex relationship testosterone shares with COVID-19.

The pro-testosterone camp hypothesizes that testosterone in COVID-19 severity is related to its effect on the cytokine storm. Studies show that testosterone downregulates inflammation and biomarkers including interleukin-6, or IL-6. In fact, a low testosterone level from hypogonadism, unhealthy aging, or coronary artery disease generates a pro-inflammatory state. However, treating

COVID-19 patients with testosterone poses significant risks, mainly due to the association of exogenous sex hormone supplementation with a hypercoagulable state that significantly increases the risk of stroke and blood clots. And as we know, severe COVID-19 in and of itself, is a pro-clotting state. Therefore, supplemental testosterone in this setting may be an especially dangerous combination outside of clinical trial or hospital setting. Moreover, the clinical utility of measuring testosterone levels is unclear given uncertain management of abnormal values that may be discovered.

And then, there is the anti-testosterone camp[177]. Androgens are male hormones that include testosterone. The production of a protein called transmembrane protein serine 2, or TMPRSS2, is dependent on the androgen receptor. TMPRSS2 augments viral entry, viral invasion, and virulence. TMPRSS2 and its family members also activate Spike, which as you know is the enhancer of the ACE receptor responsible for viral virulence. This information has prompted studies on ACE and TMPRSS2 variants in large cohorts of COVID-19 patients. Like ACE, TMPRSS2 is produced in the lungs making the use of TMPRSS2 inhibitors, currently used in prostate cancer, a potential treatment in severe COVID-19. Testosterone's effect on TMPRSS2 production may indeed play a central role in the male-predominant severity of COVID-19. Moreover, the hyper-androgenic (over-*testosterone*-ated) profile of some young men could partly explain the severe course of COVID-19 a subset of young men inexplicably experience.

YOUTH, KAWASAKI & COVID TOES

Aside from the role of testosterone in a small cohort of young men with COVID-19, the profile of youth uniquely affected by COVID-19 is unclear aside from the general risk factor profiles of a compromised immune system et cetera. An alarming manifestation of COVID-19 in children and young adults that has received substantial media attention is multisystem inflammatory syndrome, or MIS. MIS of often compared to characteristics of Kawasaki disease (KD), toxic shock syndrome (TSS), and adult COVID-19[178,179,180].

Kawasaki disease is an immune system disorder in younger people that causes inflammation of the blood vessels, or vasculitis, associated with skin rash and a red, swollen tongue. Toxic shock syndrome is a fulminant inflammatory response to a foreign body and mentioned on the back of every tampon box as a warning to young women. The common thread between MIS, KD, and TSS is immune system dysfunction and a supped up pro-inflammatory state. As you know, severe COVID-19 disease in the adult is defined by the catastrophic cytokine storming of a defunct immune system and a chaotic pro-inflammatory response, which is eerily similar to MIS in children. Why then, do they present differently? The truth is, they presently more similarly than we think and treated in a nearly identical manner.

Children with MIS most commonly present with fever, conjunctivitis, gastrointestinal symptoms, and rash. They may have persistently elevated inflammatory markers like IL-6 (ring a bell?), elevated pro-clotting biomarkers such a D-dimer, and, rarely, shock, cardiac injury, and the formation of coronary artery aneurysms indirectly related to unmitigated IL-6[181]. Adults with severe COVID-19 present similarly with the exception of more predominant lung and kidney dysfunction. One hypothesis is that children have lower levels of ACE in the lungs[182], leading to less pronounced respiratory symptoms. However, management of both diseases includes immune system modulators, antibody treatments, and/or supportive care[183]. An interesting and potentially important difference is the timing of presentation in adults versus children. So far, most children seem to have developed symptoms of MIS after the COVID-19 peak, have antibodies signifying prior exposure, and may not be positive for active infection. This suggests maladaptive post-exposure immunity in children whose immune systems are less mature than healthy adults.

Perhaps no other finding highlights the similarities between the severe, adult form of COVID-19 and pediatric MIS than dermatological stigmata[184,185]. An immune-inflammatory Kawasaki-like rash is pathognomonic of MIS in children. Similarly, immune-inflammatory dermatological abnormalities occur in adult forms of COVID-19, ergo the infamous COVID toes. In a similar fashion to how diseases with dermatological signs that affect both adults and children present, they are treated similarly too. In the case of COVID-19, off-label use of steroids and medications that dilate blood vessels in the extremities such as calcium channel blockers are proposed.

COVID toes, scientifically referred to as pseudo-chilblains (pseudo-frostbite), albeit catchy, is not the only dermatological manifestation of COVID-19. There are also maculopapular eruptions (dengue-like sandpaper rash), vesicular eruptions (measles and chickenpox-like lesions), urticarial (hives), and livedo or necrosis ('reptile' pattern or sloughing). These findings most commonly occur in middle-aged adults and precede or align with symptom onset. Livedo and necrosis are associated with the poorest prognosis, and COVID toes that manifest after symptom onset are associated with milder disease course and younger age.

AGE, PROTOPLASM & METABOLISM IN IMMUNITY

The CDC designated age greater than 65 to be the highest risk age group[186]. Although biological and functional age do not always correlate, this is a fair, albeit rough estimate. The immune system simply becomes less active as we age, hence why the overactive immune systems of people with autoimmune disease in their youth and middle age become less aggressive in older age, often justifying cessation of immunosuppressive treatment. This is known as immunosenescence, or immune system senility. Unfortunately, immunosenescent people frequently live in close proximity, such as in a nursing home setting, where some of the most serious outbreaks of COVID-19 have occurred[187].

People of any age with a compromised immune system are at risk for a more serious course of COVID-19 as well[188]. This includes cancer, cancer treatment, bone marrow or organ transplantation, anti-transplant rejection medications, autoimmune disease, medications for autoimmune disease, other chronic immunosuppressive agents, genetic or acquired immune deficiencies, and poorly controlled HIV or AIDS. This also applies to people chronically taking medications like hydroxychloroquine or antibody therapies for diseases such as lupus and rheumatoid arthritis. In these cases, higher risk of contracting COVID-19 is dependent on the underlying disease and the immunosuppressive effect of *long-term* use of these medications. Although the anti-inflammatory properties of steroids are beneficial in opposing COVID-19's cytokine storm, chronic, daily use of steroids weakens the immune system, impairs endogenous steroid production, and creates dependency on exogenous steroids for important body functions. This is not relevant to short-term use of steroids for diseases such as COVID-19.

Moreover, poorly controlled diabetes is synonymous with an immunocompromised state. Chronic hyperglycemia, or high blood sugar, slows blood flow leading to poorly perfused areas more prone to injury and less able to heal. The healing process is often undercut by superimposed infection, which the poorly controlled diabetic is ill-equip to fix. Hyperglycemia increases cellular levels of calcium, which in turn reduces ATP needed to perform important energy-expending functions including viral phagocytosis (elimination via gulping). In addition to impeding phagocytosis, leukocytes (first-line immune system cells) are unable to mobilize to sites of infection and initiate programmed cell death of tissues that are a liability to viable cells.

Hyperglycemia also impairs the immune system's complement function (triage team), limits the production of neutrophils (extermination and cleaning crew), and is associated with a chronic state of acid-base imbalance. In COVID-19, poorly controlled diabetics' poor blood flow, increased risk of superimposed bacterial infection, poor energy utilization, and suboptimal clearance of pathogens put them at higher risk for the development of severe COVID-19. There is also mounting evidence that COVID-19 may precipitate insulin resistance in susceptible people[189].

LUNGS, OBESITY & THE SKINNY-FAT PARADOX

Severe obesity (BMI >40) is a risk factor for a more severe course of COVID-19. Some camps harp on anecdotal evidence that plays devil's advocate for the obesity survival paradox[190]. This is attributed to non-specific factors such as increased 'reserves' in obese people and the presence of metabolic syndrome in non-obese counterparts (the skinny-fat paradox). Several studies describe a more severe course of COVID-19 pneumonia is obese patients, comparable to increased age in many cases[191]. Structurally, this is related to impaired respiratory mechanics and gas exchange, increased airway resistance, low lung volumes because of increased intra-abdominal girth, and poor respiratory muscle strength. Recent studies show that even overweight individuals with a BMI >30 are at higher risk for contracting COVID-19 independent of age, sex, and other risk factors[192].

Obese people also have increased prevalence of obstructive sleep apnea, or OSA[193]. Both obese and non-obese people with chronic lung disease and moderate to severe asthma are at risk for a more serious course of COVID-19 because of decreased lung capacity and peak oxygen efficiency, especially in COPD[194] and OSA. People with COPD and OSA may have a lower oxygen sensor threshold with baseline oxygen levels of 88 to 93% rather than the 'normal' 96 to 100%. Their lungs and bodies are chronically, mildly deprived of oxygen making the insult of an acute disease that induces oxygen deprivation more serious. The ACE receptor for SARS-CoV-2 is also more heavily concentrated in diseased lungs and in chronic smokers, whether they have COPD or subclinical lung disease.

Obese and non-obese people are also affected by cardiovascular diseases such as hypertension and hyperlipidemia (high cholesterol), which increases risk of severe COVID-19 via different mechanisms[195]. If you remember the renin-angiotensin-aldosterone, or RAAS, system as it relates to ACE, hypertension leads to dysfunction of the RAAS system. Chronic hypertension and hyperlipidemia generate a chronic level inflammation that makes an acute inflammatory insult such as COVID-19 result in a more fulminant disease course. In obese people, however, it is the heightened interplay of metabolic syndrome (hyperglycemia, hypertension, and hyperlipidemia) and greater incidence of comorbidities such as cardiovascular disease, lung disease, and kidney disease that increases overall risk of severe COVID-19.

For a multitude of reasons, obese and non-obese minorities such a black and Hispanic people are disproportionately affected by COVID-19. Recent studies suggest that increased incidence of COVID-19 in minorities is not directly related to cardiovascular, metabolic, socioeconomic, or vitamin D status[196]. However, subtle yet significant differences in access to *good* healthcare and healthy literacy may not accurately be reflected in standard public health metrics. And unfortunately, public health metrics also suboptimally 'size up' the psychosocial effects COVID-19 has on minorities, the majority, and everyone in between.

XIII. PSYCHOLOGICAL WARFARE
SURVIVAL OF THE WELL-ADJUSTED

Out of every one hundred men, ten shouldn't even be there, eighty are just targets, nine are the real fighters, and we are lucky to have them, for they make the battle. Ah, but the one, one is a warrior, and he will bring the others back.

—Heraclitus
  Greek Process Philosopher, Material Monist, Metaphysician & Forefather of Logic

The COVID-19 pandemic has manufactured a new status quo that is unsettling to most, unearthed the best in a few, and unveiled the worst in some. I personally will not forget a glaring example of the latter. A *very* elderly woman in a diaper that smelled of urine and feces had slipped out of her wheelchair and was crying for help on the cold linoleum floor. After feebly trying to help his mother, her elderly, disabled son looked up and around for a helping hand, which fell on blind eyes and deaf ears in the middle of a busy clinic waiting room.

I was multitasking and distracted. Now that I was out of the COVID-19 ICU, my N-95 was MIA. My flimsy paper mask was falling off as I ran around coordinating labs and testing for our COVID-19 clinical trial. Our research nurse, Briana, pointed out the woman on the floor. I surveyed my surroundings to try and piece together how an elderly woman crying for help had not been assisted in a room full of able-bodied, unoccupied people impatiently waiting and complaining. Briana then looked at me with defeated eyes. She whispered "Farah, someone just walked by, stared at that old lady, and literally said *I'm going to pretend I didn't see that*, covered her eyes, and roadrunner-ed out of here." Before Briana had time to find gloves and PPE, I was down on the floor, elbows-to-armpits and face-to-face with the woman to hoist her up into her wheelchair. Briana looked at me half-heartedly relieved and partially worried. The receptionist then warned me to be careful because the woman was a COVID-19 'rule out.' I shooed away the knee-jerk reaction to retreat and proceeded to check the woman and her son out for any obvious injury, both mental and physical. As they made their way out of the waiting room, I looked around at my fellow human cohorts: embarrassed, indifferent, self-involved. And, for just a moment, my unwavering faith in humanity wavered. Luckily, just as fate was on my side after two-and-a-half months on the COVID-19 ICU frontlines, I again tested negative a week or so later.

Although a dramatic example such as this reaffirms the obvious, it pales in comparison to the daily breaches of human decency somehow made excusable by petty annoyances and surmountable stressors people face in the current pandemic. And so, in an attempt to restore faith in humanity, we will examine the psychological warfare all around us by applying a few tenets from the principles of military psychology[197].

TERRORISM

Although acts of terror cause chaos and even the word evokes a sense of uneasiness in most, terrorism and the terrorist are usually organized and strategic with a well-developed, albeit inflexible, anti-establishment ideology. The terrorist and acts of terror that are unstable are a liability and do not instill confidence in potential prospects and recruits. However, even the most cunning terrorist psyche is a fragile house of cards in the guise of superiority that exploits the deepest fears and need for belonging in the equally fragile psyches of others.

While SARS-CoV-2 is a virulent pathogen and a terrorist in the bodies of an unfortunate few, the true terrorists are the socioeconomic and biopsychosocial entities manipulating us through the iron curtain. Relentless regurgitation of conflicting information and reactionary implementation of rules that appear helter-skelter may indeed have an underlying agenda. And, with some exception, non-stop, sensationalized media coverage serves as a sort of 'popular culture' terrorism. Regardless of credibility, this propaganda strongly influences people from all sects of society, whether by reinforcing a 'sheeple'-esque herd mentality in one or planting a seed in the educated, speculative mind of another. On the other hand, unhinged conspiracy theorists, zealots, rioters, and fear-mongers remain on the fringes of society with neither lasting impact nor meaningful influence beyond their 15 minutes.

OPERATIONAL & TACTICAL PSYCHOLOGY

Operational psychology serves to influence people to voluntary or involuntarily engage in objectives of societal interest through the use of strategies from profiling to interrogation. COVID-19 mitigation strategies are based on operational psychology, some of which are voluntary but most of which are 'socially' mandated. Tactical psychology takes a deep dive into how people interact with the enemy by using psychological techniques and historical patterns. The goal is to identify tactics to *avoid* fighting at all costs. Re-opening strategies in the aftermath of COVID-19 and planning for future waves employ tactical psychology. As such, mitigation techniques, re-opening strategies, and contingency plans have greatly impacted humankind at large.

In the case of COVID-19 mitigation and re-opening strategies, if one considers 'profiling' as a means of understanding a cohort of interest to facilitate compliance of a proposed objective, then countries like the US have failed. This is because blanket statements and generic rules do not homogenously assimilate in a heterogeneous climate, neither pre- nor post-COVID-19. Often, misaligned goals and objectives lead to televised circus-like interrogations and adjudication of blame. A mildly idealistic, yet doable, goal would be a centralized infrastructure that delegates state- and demographic-specific techniques to fluidly implement mitigation and re-opening strategies to yield more effective and sustainable results now and in the future.

DEFENSE MECHANISMS

Even for the educated citizen, terrorism compromises our sense of safety and impedes upon our ability to adjust during a challenging time such as the COVID-19 pandemic. Unhealthy defense mechanisms[198] such as regression into a state of helplessness or repression into a state of blissful ignorance are easier default modes than perseverance for the sake of self-preservation and unified adaptation. In the rare circumstance that even physiological needs are not met, in pockets of the developed world or in the developing world, overcoming the unhealthy survival instincts of misguided anger, foolish bargaining, primitive aggression, and risk-taking behavior presents an even greater challenge.

For people dependent on a sense of love and belonging[199,200], social isolation and distancing may precipitate depressed mood and dissociation from sense of self. Defense mechanisms such as introjection, or conforming feelings for approval, result in bending and breaking to accommodate for every 'fact' and frame of reference into one's COVID-19 'worldview.' The use of projection and splitting, or seeing one's faults in others, may then be discriminately used against voices of reasons that do not align with those who provide love and a sense of belonging. At the other end of the spectrum, for people who are independent and value a sense of autonomy, quarantine and threats to 'free-will' evoke a sense of anxiety and rebellion. Defense mechanisms such as rationalization (excusing and justifying mistakes) or denial (refusing to face negative behavior) result in rebelling against or neglecting mitigation strategies or ridiculing and labeling those who choose to.

For people dependent on attention and validation, the COVID-19 pandemic has mixed effects[201]. Many with a resilient sense of belonging, purpose, and esteem have demonstrated genuine empathy, respect, and action for something greater than themselves. Others have used the defense mechanism of compensation in flexing an existing strength to hide glaring disconnect. Some have used reaction formation by showcasing that they are different than their peers without engaging in tangible, effectual change. In the riots following the first wave of COVID-19, the commonly used defense mechanism of introjection, whereby many privileged people took a 'stand' against a gross injustice, was exposed when misguided public outcry dissented into their purview.

Similar defense mechanisms are used by people whose sense of esteem has been compromised by recent COVID-19-related unemployment[202]. These people may displace their frustrations on an easy target such as family or vulnerable strangers rather than the perpetrator, who may be a source of fear and intimation or simply be inaccessible or intangible. A healthier defense mechanism is identification. By attaching to something positive, such as a cause or movement they are attracted to, people can temporarily 'siphon' esteem. However, if the cause or movement is a superficial investment without direct involvement, this esteem is short-lived and fleeting. For essential workers, from grocery store clerks to those in environmental services, to whom greater responsibility is delegated and more commendation given than pre-COVID-19, interpretations of these changes vary[203]. For some, their sense of esteem and belonging may grow whereas others may feel unsafe and involuntarily forced into a position with more expectations than they signed up for.

Perhaps no other COVID-19 experience compares to that of frontline healthcare workers who carry the majority of burden in the current pandemic[204,205,206,207]. Complaints about mask-wearing, shutdowns, and other indirect, unintentional offenses from the public (the same public who give 'healthcare hero' verbal recognition and praise) coupled with AWOL essential supplies, services and resources have left the frontline healthcare worker conflicted. In rare instances, physiological and safety needs are unmet. And yet, even in these circumstances, the majority of frontliners have embraced the life instincts of social cooperation and survival. Understandably, the death instinct of reliving trauma has been an inescapable reality of the times and access to non-cookie-cutter, real-talk mental health assistance is an unmet need.

For an exceptional subset of frontliners, the pandemic has been an impetus for growth and adaptation. Through sublimation by diverting a negative perception of self and environment into an acceptable and productive outlet, these people have unmasked (no pun intended) a real-world version of self-actualization. These physicians and nurses, engrossed in a toxic environment and plagued by toxic thoughts, emergently risked life and safety for strangers and something greater than themselves. They continue to speak up and speak out against 'Big Brother' for the greater good of medicine and society.

COUNTERTERRORISM

To untether ourselves from the reigns of psychological warfare we must intellectualize, humanize, and revolutionize counterterrorism. By empowering ourselves with evidence-based information of the present, scientific principles for the future, and grounded, open minds for the unknown and unexpected, we can face the irrational times henceforth. By circumventing the survivalist dogma of 'an eye for an eye,' 'survival of the fittest,' and—insert your narcissistic mantra here—you inadvertently grace yourself with a lifeline and come to terms with an inconvenient truth. Most of us *are* the weakest links and *are* part of the thinning of the herd. And so, by ostracizing your fellow man, you are only hurting yourself. A humanistic approach to counterterrorism where an immersive look into the experiences of those both similar and far-removed from yourself, whether in your nature or not, is necessary to ensure survival of the well-adjusted and save your spot in the line of natural selection.

CLOSING REMARKS
BUILD A VAST MEMORY PALACE

The receptivity of the masses is very limited, their intelligence is small, but their *power of forgetting is enormous*. In consequence of these facts, all effective propaganda must be limited to a very few points and must harp on these in slogans until the last member of the public understands what you want him to understand by your slogan.

—Adolf Hitler
German Politician, Leader of the Nazi Party & Mass Murderer

Given the static nature inherent in any literary work and the dynamic nature of the COVID-19 pandemic, it is arbitrary to present statistics of raw numbers of cases and deaths. On the whole, it appears 80% of COVID-19 positive people in the first wave experienced a benign course, 2 to 7% experienced significant morbidity and mortality with or without hospitalization, and others lied somewhere else on the spectrum. Those who play devil's advocate and argue that low mortality is the inconsequential manifestation of 'thinning of the herd' can have the stage so long as they are as nihilistically accepting of being part of the 'thinning.' But, as human nature has demonstrated time and again, how softened the pointed tips of sharpened fingers become when the unknown encroaches upon one's own reality. Metrics are subject to change and, in and of themselves due to many uncontrolled variables, are markedly skewed in either direction. But, regardless of science, sensationalism, or sorcery, SARS-CoV-2 and COVID-19 are very real forces of profound impact, the shock waves of which, as we continue to learn, far exceeded the breadth and scope of our wildest expectations. And yet, *how easily people forget…*

Ironically, the very same people who are the first to forget happen to be those who harbor more power and influence than they know. And trust me, leaders in the field and powers that be are counting on their naivety and the power of forgetting. Instead of harnessing that power and influence, these people regress in times where there is an opportunity to rise to the occasion. They easily reconform into the mundane confines of routine that, in spite of periodically growing tired of, they covet when taken away. With greater technology and more idle time than the hunter-gatherer and *truly* surviving-epoch of our ancestors, the era of voyeurism and distraction from reality is in its element. The poor envy the rich, the rich envy the richer, and the richer envy the richest, where 'poor' and 'rich' mean the yin and yang of anything, least of all monetary. And, on the rare occasion that stars align and a gross injustice falls into the hands of a people coming back from a period of regression and a freshly lost sense of identity, the people do indeed rise up, but to what end and at what cost?

Within this small work of words on a page, I hope you decide to take the *red* pill. I hope that in 20 years all the hypotheses and theories presented here are null and void because so much progress has been made. I hope you refer to these pages far beyond their intention when seeking inspiration for your next journey. I hope you feel connected to a growing, imperfect fund of knowledge compelled to replace idol idolization of the disconnected for admiration of those who sacrifice their lives for you in spite of not knowing you; moved to contribute valuable information to passively placated passersby; and motivated to turn off the static and pass on your story to your future self over and over again to overpower the *power* of forgetting.

If we actually commit to doing so, take off the rose-colored glasses of modern life, and resist the impulse to douse fuel on anarchist-revival movements that burn out as hastily as they are lit, then and *only* then will leaders in the field and powers that be actually listen. In the case of the COVID-19 pandemic, there is a once-in-a-lifetime opportunity to learn your science and streamline your thinking to confidently trust your instincts, leave your mark, and know your enemy, even if it is looking back at you in the mirror. Until then, stay informed and see you on the other side.

BIBLIOGRAPHY

CHAPTER I

1. Jack Gilbert, Martin J. Blaser, J. Gregory Caporaso, Janet Jansson, Susan V. Lynch, Rob Knight. Current Understanding of the Human Microbiome. *Natural Medicine*, 2018; 24(4):392-400.doi:10.1038/nm.4517.
2. Fernanda Moraes, Andrea Goes. A Decade of Human Genome Project Conclusion: Scientific Diffusion About Our Genome Knowledge. *Biochemistry and Molecular Biology Education*, 2016:44(3):215-223.doi:10.1002/bmb.20952.
3. NIH Human Microbiome Portfolio Analysis Team. A Review of 10 Years of Human Microbiome Research Activities at the US National Institutes of Health, Fiscal Years 2007-2016. *Microbiome*, 2019;7(31):1-19. doi:10.1186/s40168-019-0620-y.
4. Olga Jones, Richard Seifman. Do We Need a Global Virome Project? *Lancet Global Health*, 2019;7(10): e1314-e1316.doi:10.1016/S2214-109X(19)30335-3.
5. Huihui Wang, Xuemei Li, Tao Li, Shubing Zhang, Lianzi Wang, Xian Wu, Jiaqing Liu. Genetic Sequence, Origin, and Diagnosis of SARS-CoV-2. *European Journal of Clinical Microbiology and Infectious Diseases*, 2020:1-7.doi:10.1007/s10096-020-03899-4.

CHAPTER II

6. Lewis H. Roht, Beatrice J. Selwyn, Alfonso H. Holguin. Principles of Epidemiology: A Self-Teaching Guide. Elsevier Science. Published 2013.
7. Sam Abbott, Joel Hellewell, James Munday, Sebastian Funk. The Transmissibility of Novel Coronavirus in the Early Stages of the 2019-20 Outbreak in Wuhan: Exploring Initial Point-Source Exposure Sizes and Durations Using Scenario Analysis. *Wellcome Open Research*, 2020; 5(17):1-11. doi:10.12688/wellcomeopenres.15718.1.
8. Ting Chen, Songxue Guo, Ping Zhong. Epidemic Characteristics of the COVID-19 Outbreak in Tianjin, a Well-Developed City in China. *American Journal of Infection Control*, 2020; In-Press corrected proof. doi:10.1016/j.ajic.2020.06.006.
9. Marino Gatto, Enrico Bertuzzo, Lorenzo Mari, Stefano Miccoli, Luca Carraro, Renato Casagrandi, Andrea Rinaldo. Spread and Dynamics of the COVID-19 Epidemic in Italy: Effects of Emergency Containment Measures. *Proceedings of the National Academy of Sciences of the United States of America*, 2020; 117(19):10484-10491. doi:10.1073/pnas.2004978117.
10. Hamada S Badr, Hongru Du, Maximilian Marshall, Ensheng Dong, Marietta M Squire, Lauren M Gardner. Association Between Mobility Patterns and COVID-19 Transmission in the USA: A Mathematical Modeling Study. *The Lancet: Infectious Disease*, 2020; doi:10.1016/S1473-3099(20)30553-3.

11. June-Ho Kim, Julia Ah-Reum An, Pok-kee Min, Asaf Bitton, Atul A. Gawande. How South Korea Responded to the COVID-19 Outbreak in Daegu. *New England Journal of Medicine*: Catalyst, 2020. doi:10.1056/CAT.20.0159.

12. Daniel F. Gudbjartsson, Agnar Helgason, Hakon Jonsson, Olafur T. Magnusson, Pall Melsted, Gudmundur L. Norddahl, et al. Spread of SARS-CoV-2 in the Icelandic Population. *New England Journal of Medicine*, 2020; 382:2302-2315. doi:10.1056/NEJMoa2006100.

13. Suze Wilson. Pandemic Leadership: Lessons from New Zealand's Approach to COVID-19. *Leadership*, 2020; 16(3) 279–293. doi:10.1177/1742715020929151.

14. Christer Mjåset. On Having a National Strategy in a Time of Crisis: COVID-19 Lessons from Norway. *New England Journal of Medicine: Catalyst*, 2020; doi:10.1056/CAT.20.0120.

15. David Olagniera, Trine H. Mogensena. The COVID-19 Pandemic in Denmark: Big Lessons from a Small Country. *Cytokine Growth Factor Reviews*, 2020; 53:10-12. doi:10.1016/j.cytogfr.2020.05.005.

16. Ned Stafford. COVID-19: Why Germany's Case Fatality Rate Seems So Low. *The British Medical Journal: Global Health*, 2020;369:m1395. doi:10.1136/bmj.m1395.

17. C. Jason Wang, Chun Y. Ng, Robert H. Brook. Response to COVID-19 in Taiwan: Big Data Analytics, New Technology, and Proactive Testing. *JAMA*, 2020; 323(14):1341-1342. doi:10.1001/jama.2020.3151.

18. "Immunity Passports" in the Context of COVID-19. World Health Organization. Published April 24, 2020. Accessed July 4, 2020. https://www.who.int/news-room/commentaries/detail/immunity-passports-in-the-context-of-covid-19.

19. Heba Habib. Has Sweden's Controversial COVID-19 Strategy Been Successful? *The British Medical Journal*, 2020; 369:m2376. doi:10.1136/bmj.m2376.

20. Inga Holmdahl, Caroline Buckee. Wrong But Useful—What COVID-19 Epidemiologic Models Can and Cannot Tell Us. *The New England Journal of Medicine*, 2020; doi:10.1056/NEJMp2016822.

21. Derek K. Chu, Elie A. Akl, Stephanie Duda, Karla Solo, Sally Yaacoub, Holger J. Schünemann. Physical Distancing, Face Masks, and Eye Protection to Prevent Person-to-Person Transmission of SARS-CoV-2 and COVID-19: A Systematic Review and Meta-Analysis. *The Lancet*, 2020; 395(10242):1973-1987. doi.org/10.1016/S0140-6736(20)31142-9.

22. Steffen E. Eikenberry, Marina Mancuso, Enahoro Iboi, Tin Phan, Keenan Eikenberry, Yang Kuang, et al. To Mask or Not to Mask: Modeling the Potential for Face Mask Use By the General Public to Curtail the COVID-19 Pandemic. *Infectious Disease Modeling*, 2020; 5:293-308. doi:10.1016/j.idm.2020.04.001.

CHAPTER III

23. F. Javier Ibarrondo, Jennifer A. Fulcher, David Goodman-Meza, Julie Elliott, Christian Hofmann, Mary A. Hausner, et al. Rapid Decay of Anti–SARS-CoV-2 Antibodies in Persons with Mild COVID-19. *New England Journal of Medicine*, 2020; doi:10.1056/NEJMc2025179.

24. Monica Gandhi, Deborah S. Yokoe, Diane V. Havlir. Asymptomatic Transmission: The Achilles' Heel of Current Strategies to Control COVID-19. *New England Journal of Medicine*, 2020; 382:2158-2160. doi:10.1056/NEJMe2009758.

25. Andrea Prinzi. False Negatives and Reinfections: The Challenges of SARS-CoV-2 RT-PCR Testing. American Society for Microbiology. Published April 27, 2020. Accessed June 28, 2020. https://asm.org/Articles/2020/April/False-Negatives-and-Reinfections-the-Challenges-of

26. Center for Health Security, Johns Hopkins Bloomberg School of Public Health. Serology-Based Tests for COVID-19. Accessed June 20, 2020. https://www.centerforhealthsecurity.org/resources/COVID-19/serology/Serology-based-tests-for-COVID-19.html

27. Sravanthi Parasa, Madhav Desai, Viveksandeep Thoguluva Chandrasekar. Prevalence of Gastrointestinal Symptoms and Fecal Viral Shedding in Patients With Coronavirus Disease 2019: A Systematic Review and Meta-Analysis. *JAMA Network Open*, 2020; 3(6):e2011335. doi:10.1001/jamanetworkopen.2020.11335.

28. Arno R. Bourgonje, Amaal E. Abdulle, Wim Timens, Jan-Luuk Hillebrands, Gerjan J Navis, Sanne J Gordijn, et al. Angiotensin-Converting Enzyme 2 (ACE2), SARS-CoV-2 and the Pathophysiology of Coronavirus Disease 2019 (COVID-19). *The Journal of Pathology*, 2020; 251(3):228-248. doi:10.1002/path.5471.

29. Joris R. Delanghe, Marijn M. Speeckaert, Marc L. De Buyzere. The Host's Angiotensin-Converting Enzyme Polymorphism May Explain Epidemiological Findings in COVID-19 Infections. *Clinica Chimica Acta*, 2020; 505:192-193. doi:10.1016/j.cca.2020.03.031.

30. B. Robson. COVID-19 Coronavirus Spike Protein Analysis for Synthetic Vaccines, a Peptidomimetic Antagonist, and Therapeutic Drugs, and Analysis of a Proposed Achilles' Heel Conserved Region to Minimize Probability of Escape Mutations and Drug Resistance. *Computers in Medicine and Medicine*, 2020; 121:103749. doi:10.1016/j.compbiomed.2020.103749.

31. Giuseppe Mancia, Federico Rea, Monica Ludergnani, Giovanni Apolone, Giovanni Corrao. Renin–Angiotensin–Aldosterone System Blockers and the Risk of COVID-19. *New England Journal of Medicine*, 2020; 382:2431-2440. doi:10.1056/NEJMoa2006923.

32. Mandeep R. Mehra, Sapan S. Desai, SreyRam Kuy, Timothy D. Henry, Amit N. Patel. Cardiovascular Disease, Drug Therapy, and Mortality in COVID-19. *New England Journal of Medicine*, 2020; 382:e102. doi:10.1056/NEJMoa2007621.

CHAPTER IV

33. David Ellinghaus, Frauke Degenhardt, Luis Bujanda, Maria Buti, Agustín Albillos, Pietro Invernizzi. Inflammatory Diseases and the ABO Blood Group Locus and a Chromosome 3 Gene Cluster Associated with SARS-CoV-2 Respiratory Failure in an Italian-Spanish Genome-Wide Association Analysis. *medR$_x$IV*, 2020; doi:10.1101/2020.05.31.20114991.

34. Jean M. Connors, Jerrold H. Levy. COVID-19 and Its Implications for Thrombosis and Anticoagulation. *Blood*, 2020; 135(23):2033–2040. doi:10.1182/blood.2020006000.

35. Lanying Du, Richard Y. Kao, Yusen Zhou, Yuxian He, Guangyu Zhao, Charlotte Wong, et al. Cleavage of Spike Protein of SARS Coronavirus by Protease Factor Xa is Associated with Viral Infectivity. *Biochemical and Biophysical Research Communications*, 2007; 359(1):174-179. doi:10.1016/j.bbrc.2007.05.092.

36. Taizen Nakase, Junta Moroi, Tatsuya Ishikawa. Anti-Inflammatory and Antiplatelet Effects of Non-Vitamin K Antagonist Oral Anticoagulants in Acute Phase of Ischemic Stroke Patients. *Clinical and Translational Medicine*, 2018; 17:2. doi:10.1186/s40169-017-0179-9.

37. Mariusz Kowalewski, Dario Fina, Artur Słomka, Giuseppe Maria Raffa, Gennaro Martucci, Valeria Lo Coco, et al. COVID-19 and ECMO: The Interplay Between Coagulation and Inflammation—A Narrative Review. *Critical Care*, 2020; 24(205):1-10 doi:10.1186/s13054-020-02925-3.

38. Avani R Patel, Amar R Patel, Shivank Singh, Shantanu Singh, Imran Khawaja. Applied Uses of Extracorporeal Membrane Oxygenation Therapy. *Cureus*, 2019; 11(7):e5163. doi:10.7759/cureus.5163.

39. Thomas Datzmann, Karl Träger. Extracorporeal Membrane Oxygenation and Cytokine Adsorption. *Journal of Thoracic Disease*, 2018; 10(Suppl 5):S653–S660. doi:10.21037/jtd.2017.10.128.

40. Graeme MacLaren, Dale Fisher, Daniel Brodie. Preparing for the Most Critically Ill Patients With COVID-19: The Potential Role of Extracorporeal Membrane Oxygenation *JAMA*, 2020; 323(13):1245-1246. doi:10.1001/jama.2020.2342.

41. Kollengode Ramanathan, David Antognini, Alain Combes, Matthew Paden, Bishoy Zakhary, Mark Ogino, et al. Planning and Provision of ECMO Services for Severe ARDS During the COVID-19 Pandemic and Other Outbreaks of Emerging Infectious Diseases. *Lancet*, 2020; 8(5):518-526. doi:10.1016/S2213-2600(20)30121-1.

42. Teshager Ejigu, Nikunjkumar Patel, Anuradha Sharma, Jagan Mohan Rao Vanjarapu, Vinod Nookala. Packed Red Blood Cell Transfusion as a Potential Treatment Option in COVID-19 Patients With Hypoxemic Respiratory Failure: A Case Report. *Cureus*, 2020 12(6):e8398. doi:10.7759/cureus.8398.

43. Hannelore Ehrenreich, Karin Weissenborn, Martin Begemann, Markus Busch, Eduard Vieta, Kamilla W. Miskowiak, et al. Erythropoietin as Candidate for Supportive Treatment of Severe COVID-19. *Molecular Medicine*, 2020; 26(58):1-9. doi:10.1186/s10020-020-00186-y.

44. Fabrizio Dal Moro F, Ugolino Livi. Any Possible Role of Phosphodiesterase Type 5 Inhibitors in the Treatment of Severe COVID-19 Infections? A Lesson From Urology. *Clinical Immunology*, 2020; 214:108414. doi:10.1016/j.clim.2020.108414.

CHAPTER V

45. Apoorva Mandavilli. The Coronavirus Patients Betrayed by Their Own Immune Systems. The New York Times. Published April 1, 2020. Accessed May 3, 2020. https://www.nytimes.com/2020/04/01/health/coronavirus-cytokine-storm-immune-system.html.

46. Puja Mehta, Daniel McAuley, Michael Brown, Emilie Sanchez, Rachel Tattersall, Jessica Manson. COVID-19: Consider Cytokine Storm Syndromes and Immunosuppression. *Lancet Correspondence*, 2020; doi:10.1016/ S0140-6736(20)30628-0.

47. Lili Tao, Alexandria Lowe, Guoxun Wang, Igor Dozmorov, Tyron Chang, Nan Yan, Tiffany A. Reese. Metabolic Control of Viral Infection through PPAR-α Regulation of STING Signaling. *bioR$_x$IV*. doi:10.1101/731208.

48. Hai-Yan Pan, Mihiro Yano, Hiroshi Kido. Effects of Inhibitors of Toll-Like Receptors, Protease-Activated Receptor-2 Signaling, and Trypsin on Influenza A Virus Replication and Upregulation of Cellular Factors in Cardiomyocytes. *Journal of Medical Investigation*, 2011; 58:19-28.

49. Alexander H.V. Remelsa, Wouter J.A. Derks, Berta Cillero-Pastor, Koen J.P.Verhees, Marco C. Kelders, Ward Heggermont, et al. NF-κB-Mediated Metabolic Remodeling in the Inflamed Heart in Acute Viral Myocarditis. *Biochimica et Biophysica Acta: Molecular Basis of Disease*, 2018; 1864(8):2579-2589. doi:10.1016/j.bbadis.2018.04.022

50. Aravind T. Reddy, Sowmya P. Lakshmi, Raju C. Reddy. PPARγ in Bacterial Infections: A Friend or Foe? *PPAR Research*, 2016; 7963540:1-7. doi:10.1155/2016/7963540.

51. Ishan Paranjpe, Valentin Fuster, Anuradha Lala, Adam J. Russak, Benjamin S. Glicksberg, Matthew A. Levin, et al. Association of Treatment Dose Anticoagulation With In-Hospital Survival Among Hospitalized Patients With COVID-19. *Journal of the American College of Cardiology*, 2020; 76(1):122-124. doi:10.1016/j.jacc.2020.05.001.

52. Adam Cuker, Allison Burnett, Darren Triller, Mark Crowther, Jack Ansell, Elizabeth M. Van Cott, et al. Reversal of direct oral anticoagulants: Guidance from the Anticoagulation Forum. *American Journal of Hematology*, 2019; 94(6):697-709. doi:10.1002/ajh.25475.

53. Giovanni Ponti, Monia Maccaferri, Cristel Ruini, Aldo Tomasi, Tomris Ozbend. Biomarkers Associated with COVID-19 Disease Progression. *Critical Reviews in Clinical Laboratory Sciences*, 2020:1–11.doi: 10.1080/10408363.2020.1770685.

CHAPTER VI

54. World Health Organization Model List of Essential Medications: 21st List, 2019. Accessed June 4, 2020. https://apps.who.int/iris/bitstream/handle/10665/325771/WHO-MVP-EMP-IAU-2019.06-eng.pdf?ua=1.

55. Jia Liu, Ruiyuan Cao, Mingyue Xu, Xi Wang, Huanyu Zhang, Hengrui Hu, et al. Hydroxychloroquine, a Less Toxic Derivative of Chloroquine, is Effective in Inhibiting SARS-CoV-2 Infection In Vitro. *Cell Discovery*, 2020; 6(16). doi:10.1038/s41421-020-0156-0.

56. Nathalie Costedoat-Chalumeau, Zahir Amoura, Pierre Duhaut, Du Le Thi Huong, Djame Sebbough, Bertrand Wechsler, et al. Safety of Hydroxychloroquine in Pregnant Patients with Connective Tissue Diseases: A Study of One Hundred Thirty-Three Cases Compared with a Control Group. *Arthritis and Rheumatology*, 2003; 48(11):3207-3211. doi:10.1002/art.11304.

57. Drugs and Lactation: Hydroxychloroquine. Revised April 20, 2020. Accessed May 12, 2020. https://www.ncbi.nlm.nih.gov/books/NBK501150/.

58. Plaquenil® Hydroxychloroquine Sulfate USP. Revised 2006. Accessed May 10, 2020. https://www.accessdata.fda.gov/drugsatfda_docs/label/2007/009768s041lbl.pdf.

59. Ronald Derwanda, Martin Scholzb. Does Zinc Supplementation Enhance the Clinical Efficacy of Chloroquine/Hydroxychloroquine to Win Today's Battle Against COVID-19? *Medical Hypotheses*, 2020; 142(109815). doi:10.1016/j.mehy.2020.109815.

60. Moussa Saleh, James Gabriels, David Chang, Beom Soo Kim, Amtul Mansoor, Eitezaz Mahmood, et al. Effect of Chloroquine, Hydroxychloroquine, and Azithromycin on the Corrected QT Interval in Patients With SARS-CoV-2 Infection. *Circulation: Arrhythmia and Electrophysiology*, 2020; 13(6):e008662. doi:10.1161/CIRCEP.120.008662.

61. Michael F. Marmor, Ulrich Kellner, Timothy Y.Y. Lai, Ronald B. Melles, William F. Mieler. Recommendations on Screening for Chloroquine and Hydroxychloroquine Retinopathy, *American Academy of Ophthalmology Statement*, 2016; 123(6):1386-1384. doi:10.1016/j.ophtha.2016.01.058.

62. Jeffrey K. Aronson, Nicholas DeVito, Robin E Ferner, Kamal R Mahtani, David Nunan, Annette Plüddemann. The Ethics of COVID-19 Treatment Studies: Too Many Are Open, Too Few Are Double-Masked. Center for Evidence-Based Medicine, University of Oxford. Published June 30, 2020. Accessed July 3, 2020. https://www.cebm.net/covid-19/the-ethics-of-covid-19-treatment-studies-too-many-are-open-too-few-are-double-masked/.

63. Myron S. Cohen. Hydroxychloroquine for the Prevention of COVID-19—Searching for Evidence. *New England Journal of Medicine*, 2020. doi:10.1056/NEJMe2020388.

64. Hydroxychloroquine as Chemoprevention for COVID-19 for High Risk Healthcare Workers. Published April 14, 2020. Accessed May 1, 2020. https://clinicaltrials.gov/ct2/show/NCT04345653.

65. FDA Cautions Against Use of Hydroxychloroquine or Chloroquine for COVID-19 Outside of the Hospital Setting or a Clinical Trial Due to Risk of Heart Rhythm Problems: Does Not Affect FDA-Approved Uses for Malaria, Lupus, and Rheumatoid Arthritis. Published April 24, 2020. Accessed May 1, 2020. https://www.fda.gov/drugs/drug-safety-and-availability/fda-cautions-against-use-hydroxychloroquine-or-chloroquine-covid-19-outside-hospital-setting-or.

66. Mandeep R Mehra, Sapan S Desai, Frank Ruschitzka, Amit N Patel. RETRACTED: Hydroxychloroquine or Chloroquine With or Without a Macrolide for Treatment of COVID-19: A Multinational Registry Analysis. *The Lancet*, 2020. doi:10.1016/S0140-6736(20)31180-6.

67. Heidi Ledford, Richard Van Noorden. High-Profile Coronavirus Retractions Raise Concerns About Data Oversight: Retracted Studies Had Relied on Health-Record Analyses from a Company that Declined to Share its Raw Data for an Audit. Nature. Published June 5, 2020. Accessed June 5, 2020. https://www.nature.com/articles/d41586-020-01695-w.

68. Jane Greenhalgh. Authors Retract Hydroxychloroquine Study, Citing Concern Over Data. NPR. Published June 4, 2020. Accessed June 5, 2020. https://www.npr.org/sections/coronavirus-live-updates/2020/06/04/870022834/authors-retract-hydroxychloroquine-study-citing-concern-over-data.

69. Jared S. Hopkins, Russell Gold. Hydroxychloroquine Studies Tied to Data Firm Surgisphere Retracted. The Wall Street Journal. Published June 5, 2020. Accessed June 5, 2020. https://www.wsj.com/articles/authors-retract-study-that-found-risks-of-using-antimalaria-drug-against-covid-19-11591299329.

70. Roni Caryn Rabin, Ellen Gabler. Two Huge COVID-19 Studies Are Retracted After Scientists Sound Alarms. The New York Times. Published June 4, 2020. Accessed June 5, 2020. https://www.nytimes.com/2020/06/04/health/coronavirus-hydroxychloroquine.html

CHAPTER VII

71. First FDA-Approved Vaccine for the Prevention of Ebola Virus Disease, Marking a Critical Milestone in Public Health Preparedness and Response. Published December 19, 2019. Accessed May 23, 2020. https://www.fda.gov/news-events/press-announcements/first-fda-approved-vaccine-prevention-ebola-virus-disease-marking-critical-milestone-public-health.

72. Harriet L. Robinson. HIV/AIDS Vaccines: 2018. *Clinical Pharmacology and Therapeutics*, 2018;104(6):1062–1073. doi:10.1002/cpt.1208.

73. Mark-M. Struck. Vaccine R&D Success Rates and Development Times. *Nature Biotechnology*, 1996; 14:591-593.

74. Human Challenge Trials for Vaccine Development: Regulatory Considerations. WHO Expert Committee on Biological Standardization, Geneva, Switzerland. October 17-21,

2016. Accessed April 28, 2020.
https://www.who.int/biologicals/expert_committee/Human_challenge_Trials_IK_final.pd
f.

75. Asher Mullard. COVID-19 Vaccine Development Pipeline Gears Up. *The Lancet*, 2020;
395(10239): 1751-1752. doi:10.1016/S0140-6736(20)31252-6.

76. Deborah H. Fuller, Peter Berglund. Amplifying RNA Vaccine Development. *New
England Journal of Medicine*, 2020; 382:2469-2471. doi:10.1056/NEJMcibr2009737.

77. Cormac Sheridan. Convalescent Serum Lines Up as First-Choice Treatment for
Coronavirus. *Nature Biotechnology*, 2020;38:655-658. doi:10.1038/d41587-020-00011-1.

78. John H. Beigel, Jocelyn Voell, Parag Kumar, Kanakatte Raviprakash, Hua Wu, Jin-An
Jiao, et al. Safety and Tolerability of a Novel, Polyclonal Human Anti-MERS
Coronavirus Antibody Produced from Transchromosomic Cattle: A Phase 1 Randomized,
Double-Blind, Single-Dose-Escalation Study. *The Lancet: Infectious Diseases*, 2020;
18(4):410-418. doi:10.1016/S1473-3099(18)30002-1.

79. Vaccines Licensed for Use in the United States. Food and Drug Administration. Revised
April 24, 2020. Accessed May 6, 2020. https://www.fda.gov/vaccines-blood-
biologics/vaccines/vaccines-licensed-use-united-states.

80. Julie E. Ledgerwood, Theodore C. Pierson, Sarah A. Hubka, Niraj Desai, Steve Rucker,
Ingelise J. Gordon, et al. West Nile Virus DNA Vaccine Utilizing a Modified Promoter
Induces Neutralizing Antibody in Younger and Older Healthy Adults in a Phase I
Clinical Trial. *Journal of Infectious Diseases*, 2011; 203(10):1396-1404.
doi:10.1093/infdis/jir054.

81. Feng-Cai Zhu, Yu-Hua Li, Xu-Hua Guan, Li-Hua Hou, Wen-Juan Wang, Jing-Xin Li, et
al. Safety, Tolerability, and Immunogenicity of a Recombinant Adenovirus Type-5
Vectored COVID-19 Vaccine: A Dose-Escalation, Open-Label, Non-Randomized, First-
in-Human Trial. *The Lancet*, 2020; 395(10240):1845-1854. doi.org/10.1016/S0140-
6736(20)31208-3.

82. Wolfgang W. Leitner, Han Ying, Nicholas P. Restifo. DNA and RNA-Based Vaccines:
Principles, Progress, and Prospects. *Vaccine*, 1999; 18(9-10):765–777.

83. Arthur A. Vandenbark, Nicole E. Culbertson, Richard M. Bartholomew, Jianya Huan,
Marci Agotsch, Dorian LaTocha, et al. Therapeutic Vaccination with a Trivalent T-Cell
Receptor (TCR) Peptide Vaccine Restores Deficient FoxP3 Expression and TCR
Recognition in Subjects with Multiple Sclerosis. *Immunology*, 2008; 123(1):66–78.
doi:10.1111/j.1365-2567.2007.02703.x.

84. Danuta Gutowska-Owsiak, Graham S. Ogg. Therapeutic Vaccines for Allergic Disease.
NPJ Vaccines, 2017; 2(12). doi:10.1038/s41541-017-0014-8.

85. Ensuring the Safety of Vaccines in the United States. Food and Drug Administration.
Revised January 2018. Accessed July 1, 2020.
https://www.cdc.gov/vaccines/hcp/conversations/downloads/vacsafe-ensuring-color-
office.pdf.

CHAPTER VIII

86. WHO Welcomes Preliminary Results About Dexamethasone Use in Treating Critically Ill COVID-19 Patients. Published June 16, 2020. Accessed June 20, 2020. https://www.who.int/news-room/detail/16-06-2020-who-welcomes-preliminary-results-about-dexamethasone-use-in-treating-critically-ill-covid-19-patients.

87. Efficacy and Safety of Corticosteroids in COVID-19. Published February 18, 2020. Accessed May 3, 2020. https://clinicaltrials.gov/ct2/show/NCT04273321.

88. Targeted Steroids for ARDS Due to COVID-19 Pneumonia: A Pilot Randomized Clinical Trial. Published April 24, 2020. Accessed May 14, 2020. https://clinicaltrials.gov/ct2/show/NCT04360876.

89. Richard T. Eastman, Jacob S. Roth, Kyle R. Brimacombe, Anton Simeonov, Min Shen, Samarjit Patnaik, et al. Remdesivir: A Review of Its Discovery and Development Leading to Emergency Use Authorization for Treatment of COVID-19. *ACS Central Science*, 2020; 6(5):672–683. doi:10.1021/acscentsci.0c00489.

90. Timothy P. Sheahan, Amy C. Sims, Sarah R. Leist, Alexandra Schäfer, John Won, Ariane J. Brown, et al. Comparative Therapeutic Efficacy of Remdesivir and Combination Lopinavir, Ritonavir, and Interferon Beta Against MERS-CoV. *Nature Communications*, 2020; 11(222); doi:10.1038/s41467-019-13940-6.

91. Remdesivir Emergency Use Authorization Letter. Published May 1, 2020. Accessed June 1, 2020. https://www.fda.gov/media/137564/download.

92. Meagan L. Adamsick, Ronak G. Gandhi, Monique R. Bidell, Ramy H. Elshaboury, Roby P. Bhattacharyya, Arthur Y. Kim, et al. Remdesivir in Patients with Acute or Chronic Kidney Disease and COVID-19. *Journal of the American Society of Nephrology*, 2020; 31(7):1384-1386. doi:10.1681/ASN.2020050589.https://jasn.asnjournals.org/content/31/7/1384.

93. John H. Beigel, Kay M. Tomashek, Lori E. Dodd, Aneesh K. Mehta, Barry S. Zingman, Andre C. Kalil, et al. Remdesivir for the Treatment of COVID-19—Preliminary Report. *New England Journal of Medicine*, 2020. doi:10.1056/NEJMoa2007764.

94. Grant S. Schulert. Can Tocilizumab Calm the Cytokine Storm of COVID-19? *The Lancet*, 2020; doi:10.1016/S2665-9913(20)30210-1.

95. Xiaoling Xu, Mingfeng Han, Tiantian Li, Wei Sun, Dongsheng Wang, Binqing Fu, et al. Effective Treatment of Severe COVID-19 Patients with Tocilizumab. *Proceedings of the National Academy of Sciences of the United States of America*, 2020; 117(20): 10970–10975. doi:10.1073/pnas.2005615117.

96. ACTEMRA (tocilizumab) Food and Drug Administration. Revised August 2017. Accessed May 1, 2020. https://www.accessdata.fda.gov/drugsatfda_docs/label/2017/125276s114lbl.pdf.

97. Susanna K. P. Lau, Candy C. Y. Lau, Kwok-Hung Chan, Clara P. Y. Li, Honglin Chen, Dong-Yan Jin, et al. Delayed Induction of Proinflammatory Cytokines and Suppression of Innate Antiviral Response by the Novel Middle East Respiratory Syndrome

Coronavirus: Implications for Pathogenesis and Treatment. *Journal of General Virology*, 2013; 94(12). doi.org/10.1099/vir.0.055533-0.

98. Tocilizumab in COVID-19 Pneumonia (TOCIVID-19). Published March 20, 2020. Accessed April 15, 2020. https://clinicaltrials.gov/ct2/show/NCT04317092.

99. A Study to Evaluate the Safety and Efficacy of Tocilizumab in Patients With Severe COVID-19 Pneumonia (COVACTA). Published March 25, 2020. Accessed April 20, 2020. https://clinicaltrials.gov/ct2/show/NCT04320615.

100. Tocilizumab in the Treatment of Coronavirus Induced Disease (COVID-19) (CORON-ACT). Published April 6, 2020. Accessed April 20, 2020. https://clinicaltrials.gov/ct2/show/NCT04335071.

101. Akram Khan, Cody Benthin, Brian Zeno, Timothy E. Albertson, John Boyd, Jason D. Christie, et al. A Pilot Clinical Trial of Recombinant Human Angiotensin-Converting Enzyme 2 in Acute Respiratory Distress Syndrome. *Critical Care*, 2017; 21(234). doi:10.1186/s13054-017-1823-x.

102. Marc Feldmann, Ravinder N Maini, James N Woody, Stephen T Holgate, Gregory Winter, Matthew Rowland, et al. Trials of Anti-Tumor Necrosis Factor Therapy for COVID-19 are Urgently Needed. *The Lancet*, 2020; 395(10234):1407-1409. doi:10.1016/S0140-6736(20)30858-8.

103. Haibo Zhang, Josef M. Penninger, Yimin Li, Nanshan Zhong, Arthur S. Slutsky. Angiotensin-Converting Enzyme 2 (ACE2) as a SARS-CoV-2 Receptor: Molecular Mechanisms and Potential Therapeutic Target. *Intensive Care Medicine*, 2020; 46:586–590. doi:10.1007/s00134-020-05985-9.

104. Recombinant Human Angiotensin-Converting Enzyme 2 (rhACE2) as a Treatment for Patients With COVID-19. Published February 27, 2020. Accessed June 1, 2020. https://clinicaltrials.gov/ct2/show/NCT04287686

105. Neda Roshanravan, Samad Ghaffari, Mehdi Hedayatib. Angiotensin Converting Enzyme-2 as Therapeutic Target in COVID-19. *Diabetes and Metabolic Syndrome: Clinical Research and Reviews*, 2020; 14(4):637-639. doi:10.1016/j.dsx.2020.05.022.

106. Giuseppe Marano, Stefania Vaglio, Simonetta Pupella, Giuseppina Facco, Liviana Catalano, Giancarlo M. Liumbruno, Giuliano Grazzini. Convalescent Plasma: New Evidence for an Old Therapeutic Tool? *Blood Transfusion*, 2016; 14(2):152-157. doi:10.2450/2015.0131-15.

107. Thomas C. Luke, Arturo Casadevall, Stanley J. Watowich, Stephen L. Hoffman, John H. Beigel, Timothy H. Burgess. Hark Back: Passive Immunotherapy for Influenza and Other Serious Infections. *Critical Care Medicine*, 2010; 38(4):e66-e73. doi:10.1097/CCM.0b013e3181d44c1e.

108. Qian Zhao, Yong He. Challenges of Convalescent Plasma Therapy on COVID-19. *Journal of Clinical Virology*, 2020; 127:104358. doi:10.1016/j.jcv.2020.104358.

109. Pierre Tiberghien, Xavier de Lambalerie, Pascal Morel, Pierre Gallian, Karine Lacombe, Yazdan Yazdanpanah. Collecting and Evaluating Convalescent Plasma for

COVID-19 Treatment: Why and How. *Sociedad Argentina de Hematología*, 2020. doi:10.1111/vox.12926.

110.   Arturo Casadevall, Michael J. Joyner, Liise-Anne Pirofski. A Randomized Trial of Convalescent Plasma for COVID-19—Potentially Hopeful Signals. *JAMA*, 2020. doi:10.1001/jama.2020.10218.

111.   Koduri Sridevi, Amit Munjal, Ajay Chandran, S. Nachiappan, Praveena Raman, Sukriti Bhalla, et al. Convalescent Plasma Therapy for Prophylaxis and Treatment of COVID-19: A Systematic Research of Facts and Files, A Narrative Review. *Annals of Clinical and Laboratory Research*, 2020; 8(2):314. doi:10.36648/2386-5180.8.2.314.

112.   Human Convalescent Plasma for High Risk Children Exposed or Infected With SARS-CoV-2 (COVID-19). Published May 6, 2020. Accessed June 1, 2020. https://clinicaltrials.gov/ct2/show/NCT04377672.

113.   COVIDPlasma.org, an AABB Initiative. Accessed May 3, 2020. https://covidplasma.org/.

114.   Donate COVID-19 Plasma. Food and Drug Administration. Accessed May 2, 2020. https://www.fda.gov/emergency-preparedness-and-response/coronavirus-disease-2019-covid-19/donate-covid-19-plasma.

115.   Expanded Access to Convalescent Plasma for the Treatment of Patients With COVID-19. ClinicalTrials.gov Identifier: NCT04338360. Published April 8, 2020. Accessed May 1, 2020. https://www.uscovidplasma.org/.

CHAPTER IX

116.   Rüdiger Hardeland. Melatonin and the Theories of Aging: A Critical Appraisal of Melatonin's Role in Anti-Aging Mechanisms. *Journal of Pineal Research*, 2013; 55:325-356. doi:10.1111/jpi.12090.

117.   Rui Zhang, Xuebin Wang, Leng Ni, Xiao Di, Baitao Ma, Shuai Niu, et al. COVID-19: Melatonin as a Potential Adjuvant Treatment. *Life Sciences*, 2020; 250:117583. doi:10.1016/j.lfs.2020.117583.

118.   George Anderson, Moses Rodriguez. Multiple Sclerosis: The Role of Melatonin and N-acetylserotonin. *Multiple Sclerosis and Related Disorders*, 2015; 4:112-123. doi:10.1016/j.msard.2014.12.001.

119.   Ciaran J. McMullan, Eva S. Schernhammer, Eric B. Rimm, Frank B. Hu, John P. Forman. Melatonin Secretion and the Incidence of Type 2 Diabetes. *JAMA*, 2013; 309(13):1388–1396. doi:10.1001/jama.2013.2710.

120.   Souvik Maitra, Dalim Kumar Baidya, Puneet Khanna. Melatonin in Perioperative Medicine: Current Perspective. *Saudi Journal of Anesthesia*, 2013; 7(3):315-321. doi:10.4103/1658-354X.115316.

121.   Zukiswa Jiki, Sandrine Lecour, Frederic Nduhirabandi. Cardiovascular Benefits of Dietary Melatonin: A Myth or a Reality? *Frontiers in Physiology*, 2018; 9:528. doi:10.3389/fphys.2018.00528.

122.	Maria Permuy, Mónica López-Peña, Antonio González-Cantalapiedra, Fernando Muñoz. Melatonin: A Review of Its Potential Functions and Effects on Dental Diseases. *International Journal of Molecular Sciences*, 2017; 18(4):865. doi:10.3390/ijms18040865.

123.	Margarita R. Ramis, Susana Estebana, Antonio Mirallesa, Dun-Xian Tan, Russel J. Reiterb. Caloric Restriction, Resveratrol and Melatonin: Role of SIRT1 and Implications for Aging and Related-Diseases. *Mechanisms of Aging and Development*, 2015; 146–148:28-41. doi:10.1016/j.mad.2015.03.008.

124.	Linli Yao, Pengfei Lu, Eng-Ang Ling. Melatonin Suppresses Toll Like Receptor 4-Dependent Caspase-3 Signaling Activation Coupled with Reduced Production of Proinflammatory Mediators in Hypoxic Microglia. *PLoS One*, 2016; 11(11):e0166010. doi:10.1371/journal.pone.0166010.

125.	Gaia Favero, Lorenzo Franceschetti, Francesca Bonomini, Luigi Fabrizio Rodella, Rita Rezzani. Melatonin as an Anti-Inflammatory Agent Modulating Inflammasome Activation. *International Journal of Endocrinology*, 2017; doi:10.1155/2017/1835195.

126.	Shing-Hwa Huang, Ching-Len Liao, Shyi-Jou Chend, Li-Ge Shi, Li Lin, Yuan-Wu Chen, et al. Melatonin Possesses an Anti-Influenza Potential Through Its Immune Modulatory Effect. *Journal of Functional Foods*, 2019; 58:189-198. doi:10.1016/j.jff.2019.04.062.

127.	Michela Silvestri, Giovanni A Rossi. Melatonin: Its Possible Role in the Management of Viral Infections: A Brief Review. *Italian Journal of Pediatrics*, 2013;39:61. doi:10.1186/1824-7288-39-61.

128.	Wei Hu, Chao Deng, Zhiqiang Ma, Dongjin Wang, Chongxi Fan, Tian Li, et al. Utilizing Melatonin to Combat Bacterial Infections and Septic Injury. *British Journal of Pharmacology*, 2017; 174(9):754–768. doi:10.1111/bph.13751.

129.	Hui-Mei Wu, Cui-Cui Zhao, Qiu-Meng Xie, Juan Xu, Guang-He Fei. TLR2-Melatonin Feedback Loop Regulates the Activation of NLRP3 Inflammasome in Murine Allergic Airway Inflammation. *Frontiers in Immunology*, 2020. doi:10.3389/fimmu.2020.00172.

130.	Geng-Chin Wu, Chung-Kan Peng, Wen-I Liao, Hsin-Ping Pao, Kun-Lun Huang, Shi-Jye Chu. Melatonin Receptor Agonist Protects Against Acute Lung Injury Induced By Ventilator Through Up-Regulation of IL-10 Production. *Respiratory Research*, 2020; 21(65). doi:10.1186/s12931-020-1325-2.

131.	B. S. Alghamdi. The Neuroprotective Role of Melatonin in Neurological Disorders. *Journal of Neuroscience Research*, 2018; 96(7):1136–1149. doi:10.1002/jnr.24220.

132.	SR Lewis, MW Pritchard, OJ Schofield-Robinson, P. Alderson, AF Smith. Melatonin for the Promotion of Sleep in Adults in the Intensive Care Unit. *Cochrane Database of Systematic Reviews*, 2018; 5(CD012455). doi:10.1002/14651858.CD012455.pub2.

133.	Russel J. Reiter, Pedro Abreu-Gonzalez, Paul E. Marik, Alberto Dominguez-Rodriguez. Therapeutic Algorithm for Use of Melatonin in Patients With COVID-19. *Frontiers in Medicine*, 2020. doi:10.3389/fmed.2020.00226.

134.	Irene García García, Miguel Rodriguez-Rubio, Amelia Rodríguez Mariblanca, Lucía Martínez de Soto, Lucía Díaz García, Jaime Monserrat Villatoro, et al. A Randomized Multicenter Clinical Trial to Evaluate the Efficacy of Melatonin in the Prophylaxis of SARS-CoV-2 Infection in High-Risk Contacts (MeCOVID Trial): A Structured Summary of a Study Protocol for a Randomized Controlled Trial. *Trials*, 2020; 21.466. doi:10.1186/s13063-020-04436-6(2020).

135.	Ali Daneshkhah, Vasundhara Agrawal, Adam Eshein, Hariharan Subramanian, Hemant Kumar Roy, Vadim Backman. The Possible Role of Vitamin D in Suppressing Cytokine Storm and Associated Mortality in COVID-19 Patients. *medR$_x$IV*, 2020. doi:10.1101/2020.04.08.20058578.

136.	Ainoosh Golpour, Stefan Bereswill, Markus M. Heimesaat. Antimicrobial and Immune-Modulatory Effects of Vitamin D Provide Promising Antibiotics-Independent Approaches to Tackle Bacterial Infections–Lessons Learnt from a Literature Survey. European *Journal of Microbiology and Immunology*, 2019; 9(3):80-87. doi:10.1556/1886.2019.00014.

137.	Joseph Lee, Oliver van Hecke, Nia Roberts. Vitamin D: A Rapid Review of the Evidence for Treatment or Prevention in COVID-19. Center for Evidence-Based Medicine. Published May 1, 2020. Accessed June 3, 2020. https://www.cebm.net/covid-19/vitamin-d-a-rapid-review-of-the-evidence-for-treatment-or-prevention-in-covid-19/.

138.	M. Chakhtoura, N. Napoli, G. El Hajj Fuleihan. Myths and Facts on Vitamin D Amidst the COVID-19 Pandemic. *Metabolism*, 2020; 109:154276. doi:10.1016/j.metabol.2020.154276.

139.	Longitudinal Population-based Observational Study of COVID-19 in the UK Population (COVIDENCE UK). Published April 1, 2020. Accessed May 7, 2020. https://clinicaltrials.gov/ct2/show/NCT04330599.

140.	Anatoly V. Skalny, Lothar Rink, Olga P. Ajsuvakova, Michael Aschner, Viktor A. Gritsenko, Svetlana I. Alekseenko, et al. Zinc and Respiratory Tract Infections: Perspectives for COVID-19. *International Journal of Molecular Medicine*, 2020; 46(1):17-26. doi:10.3892/ijmm.2020.4575.

141.	Amit Kumar, Yuichi Kubota, Mikhail Chernov, Hidetoshi Kasuya. Potential Role of Zinc Supplementation in Prophylaxis and Treatment of COVID-19. *Medical Hypotheses*, 2020; 109848. doi:10.1016/j.mehy.2020.109848.

142.	R. Derwanda, M. Scholzb. Does Zinc Supplementation Enhance the Clinical Efficacy of Chloroquine/Hydroxychloroquine to Win Today's Battle Against COVID-19? *Medical Hypotheses*, 2020; 142.109815. doi.org/10.1016/j.mehy.2020.109815.

143.   A Study of Hydroxychloroquine, Vitamin C, Vitamin D, and Zinc for the Prevention of COVID-19 Infection (HELPCOVID-19). Published April 6, 2020. Accessed May 1, 2020. https://clinicaltrials.gov/ct2/show/NCT04335084.

144.   Coronavirus 2019 (COVID-19)- Using Ascorbic Acid and Zinc Supplementation (COVIDAtoZ). Published April 13, 2020. Accessed May 10, 2020. https://clinicaltrials.gov/ct2/show/NCT04342728.

145.   Anitra C. Carr. Vitamin C Administration in the Critically Ill: Summary of Recent Meta-Analyses. *Critical Care*, 2019; 23(265). doi.org/10.1186/s13054-019-2538-y.

146.   Vitamin C Infusion for the Treatment of Severe 2019-nCoV Infected Pneumonia. Published February 11, 2020. Accessed April 27, 2020. https://clinicaltrials.gov/ct2/show/NCT04264533.

CHAPTER X

147.   Stephen L. Archer, Willard W. Sharp, E. Kenneth Weir. Differentiating COVID-19 Pneumonia from Acute Respiratory Distress Syndrome (ARDS) and High Altitude Pulmonary Edema (HAPE): Therapeutic Implications. *Circulation*, 2020; doi:10.1161/CIRCULATIONAHA.120.047915.

148.   Weili Han, Manhua Zhu, Jun Chen, Jing Zhang, Shengmei Zhu, Tong Li, et al. Lung Transplantation for Elderly Patients With End-Stage COVID-19 Pneumonia. *Annals of Surgery*, 2020; doi: 10.1097/SLA.0000000000003955.

149.   Alvaro Coronado Munoz, Upulie Nawaratne, David McMann, Misti Ellsworth, Jon Meliones, Konstantinos Boukas. Late-Onset Neonatal Sepsis in a Patient with COVID-19. *New England Journal of Medicine*, 2020; 382:e49. doi:10.1056/NEJMc2010614.

150.   Safiya Richardson, Jamie S. Hirsch, Mangala Narasimhan, James M. Crawford, Thomas McGinn, Karina W. Davidson. Presenting Characteristics, Comorbidities, and Outcomes Among 5700 Patients Hospitalized With COVID-19 in the New York City Area. *JAMA*, 2020; 323(20):2052-2059. doi:10.1001/jama.2020.6775.

151.   Xavier Elharrar, Youssef Trigui, Anne-Marie Dols, François Touchon, Stéphanie Martinez, Eloi Prud'homme, Laurent Papazian. Use of Prone Positioning in Nonintubated Patients With COVID-19 and Hypoxemic Acute Respiratory Failure, *JAMA*, 2020; 323(22):2336-2338. doi:10.1001/jama.2020.8255.

152.   Anna Coppo, Giacomo Bellani, Dario Winterton, Michela Di Pierro, Alessandro Soria, Paola Faverio, et al. Feasibility and Physiological Effects of Prone Positioning in Non-Intubated Patients with Acute Respiratory Failure Due to COVID-19 (PRON-COVID): A Prospective Cohort Study. *Lancet: Respiratory Medicine*, 2020; doi:10.1016/S2213-2600(20)30268-X.

153.   Claude Guérin, Jean Reignier, Jean-Christophe Richard, Pascal Beuret, Arnaud Gacouin, Thierry Boulain, et al. Prone Positioning in Severe Acute Respiratory Distress

Syndrome. *New England Journal of Medicine*, 2013; 368:2159-2168. doi:10.1056/NEJMoa1214103.

154.   Xu Li, Xiaochun Ma. Acute Respiratory Failure in COVID-19: Is It "Typical" ARDS? *Critical Care*. 2020; 24:198. doi:10.1186/s13054-020-02911-9.

155.   CF Arias, FJ Acosta, F. Bertocchini, C. Fernández-Arias. Interference of SARS-CoV-2 with the Homeostasis of Ventilation and Perfusion in the Lung. *Preprints*, 2020; doi:10.20944/preprints202005.0177.v1.

156.   Romain Barthélémy, Pierre-Louis Blot, Ambre Tiepolo, Arthur Le Galla, Claire Mayeur, Samuel Gaugain, et al. Efficacy of Almitrine in the Treatment of Hypoxemia in Sars-Cov-2 Acute Respiratory Distress Syndrome. *Chest*, 2020; doi:10.1016/j.chest.2020.05.573.

157.   Kimberly J. Dunham-Snary, Danchen Wu, Edward A. Sykes, Amar Thakrar, Leah R.G. Parlow, Jeffrey D. Mewburn, et al. Hypoxic Pulmonary Vasoconstriction: From Molecular Mechanisms to Medicine. *Chest*, 2017; 151(1):181–192. doi:10.1016/j.chest.2016.09.001.

158.   Andre Pennardt. High-Altitude Pulmonary Edema: Diagnosis, Prevention, and Treatment. *Current Sports Medicine Reports*, 2013;12(2):115-119. doi:10.1249/JSR.0b013e318287713b.

159.   Andrew M. Luks, Erik R. Swenson. COVID-19 Lung Injury and High Altitude Pulmonary Edema: A False Equation with Dangerous Implications. *Annals of the American Thoracic Society*, 2020; doi:10.1513/AnnalsATS.202004-327FR.

CHAPTER XI

160.   JP 3-07 Joint Doctrine for Military Operations Other Than War. Published June 6, 1995. Accessed July 6, 2020. https://www.bits.de/NRANEU/others/jp-doctrine/jp3_07.pdf.

161.   Alan S. Kliger, Jeffrey Silberzweig. Mitigating Risk of COVID-19 in Dialysis Facilities. *Clinical Journal of American Society of Nephrology*, 2020; 15(5):707-709. doi:10.2215/CJN.03340320.

162.   Claudio Ronco, Thiago Reis, Faeq Husain-Syed. Management of Acute Kidney Injury in Patients with COVID-19. *Lancet*, 2020; 8(7):738-742. doi:10.1016/S2213-2600(20)30229-0.

163.   Muhammad Aziz, Rawish Fatima, Wade Lee-Smith, Ragheb Assaly. The Association of Low Serum Albumin Level with Severe COVID-19: A Systematic Review and Meta-Analysis. *Critical Care*, 2020; 24:255. doi:10.1186/s13054-020-02995-3.

164.   Jian Wu, Shu Song, Hong-Cui Cao, Lan-Juan Li. Liver Diseases in COVID-19: Etiology, Treatment, and Prognosis. *World Journal of Gastroenterology*, 2020; 26(19): 2286-2293. doi:10.3748/wjg.v26.i19.2286.

165.   Shadi Yaghi, Koto Ishida, Jose Torres, Brian Mac Grory, Eytan Raz, Kelley Humbert, et al. SARS-CoV-2 and Stroke in a New York Healthcare System. *Stroke*, 2020; 51(7):2002-2011. doi:10.1161/STROKEAHA.120.030335.

166.   Gustavo C Román, Jacques Reis, Peter S Spencer, Alain Buguet, Serefnur Öztürk, Mohammad Wasay. COVID-19 International Neurological Registries. *The Lancet Correspondence*, 2020; 19:484-485.

167.   Qi Cheng, Yue Yang, Jianqun Gao. Infectivity of Human Coronavirus in the Brain. *EBioMedicine by Lancet*, 2020; 56:102799. doi:10.1016/j.ebiom.2020.102799.

168.   Karima Benameur, Ankita Agarwal, Sara C. Auld, Matthew P. Butters, Andrew S Webster, Tugba Ozturk, et al. Encephalopathy and Encephalitis Associated with Cerebrospinal Fluid Cytokine Alterations and Coronavirus Disease. *Emerging Infectious Diseases (CDC)*, 2020; 26(9). doi.org/10.3201/eid2609.202122.

169.   Takeshi Moriguchia, Norikazu Hariib, Junko Gotoa, Daiki Haradaa, Hisanori Sugawaraa, Junichi Takaminoa, et al. A First Case of Meningitis/Encephalitis Associated with SARS-Coronavirus-2. *International Journal of Infectious Diseases*, 2020; 94:55-58. doi:10.1016/j.ijid.2020.03.062.

170.   Yan-Chao Li, Wan-Zhu Bai, Tsutomu Hashikawa. The Neuroinvasive Potential of SARS-CoV2 May Play a Role in the Respiratory Failure of COVID-19 Patients. *Journal of Medical Virology*, 2020; 92(6):552-555. doi:10.1002/jmv.25728.

171.   Sonu Gandhi, Amit Kumar Srivastava, Upasana Ray, Prem Prakash Tripathi. Is the Collapse of the Respiratory Center in the Brain Responsible for Respiratory Breakdown in COVID-19 Patients? *ACS Chemical Neuroscience*, 2020; 11,1379-1381. doi:10.1021/acschemneuro.0c00217.

172.   Melanie A. Samuel, Hong Wang, Venkatraman Siddharthan, John D. Morrey, Michael S. Diamond. Axonal Transport Mediates West Nile Virus Entry into the Central Nervous System and Induces Acute Flaccid Paralysis. *Proceedings of the National Academy of Sciences of the United States of America*, 2007; 104(43):17140-17145. doi:10.1073/pnas.0705837104.

173.   Orkide O. Koyuncu, Ian B. Hogue, Lynn W. Enquist. Virus Infections in the Nervous System. *Cell Host Microbe*, 2013; 13(4):379-393. doi:10.1016/j.chom.2013.03.010.

174.   Mark A Ellul, Laura Benjamin, Bhagteshwar Singh, Suzannah Lant, Benedict Daniel Michael, Ava Easton, et al. Neurological Associations of COVID-19. *The Lancet. Neurology*, 2020; doi.org/10.1016/S1474-4422(20)30221-0.

175.   MA Topcuoglu, E Saka, SB Silverman, LH Schwamm, AB Singhal. Recrudescence of Deficits After Stroke: Clinical and Imaging Phenotype, Triggers, and Risk Factors. *JAMA Neurology*, 2017; 74(9):1048-1055. doi:10.1001/jamaneurol.2017.1668.

CHAPTER XII

176.　　　Paolo Pozzillia, Andrea Lenzib. Commentary: Testosterone, A Key Hormone in the Context of COVID-19 Pandemic. *Metabolism*, 2020; 108:154252. doi:10.1016/j.metabol.2020.154252.

177.　　　Rosanna Asselta, Elvezia Maria Paraboschi, Alberto Mantovani, Stefano Duga. ACE2 and TMPRSS2 Variants and Expression as Candidates to Sex and Country Differences in COVID-19 Severity in Italy. *medRxIV*, 2020; doi:10.1101/2020.03.30.2004787.

178.　　　Elizabeth Whittaker, Alasdair Bamford, Julia Kenny, Myrsini Kaforou, Christine E. Jones, Priyen Shah, et al. Clinical Characteristics of 58 Children With a Pediatric Inflammatory Multisystem Syndrome Temporally Associated With SARS-CoV-2. *JAMA*, 2020; doi:10.1001/jama.2020.10369.

179.　　　Lucio Verdoni, Angelo Mazza, Annalisa Gervasoni, Laura Martelli, Maurizio Ruggeri, Matteo Ciuffreda, et al. An Outbreak of Severe Kawasaki-Like Disease at the Italian Epicenter of the SARS-CoV-2 Epidemic: An Observational Cohort Study. *The Lancet*, 2020; 395(10239):1771-1778. doi:10.1016/S0140-6736(20)31103-X.

180.　　　Elizabeth Barnett Pathak, Jason L. Salemi, Natasha Sobers, Janelle Menard, Ian R. Hambleton. COVID-19 in Children in the United States: Intensive Care Admissions, Estimated Total Infected, and Projected Numbers of Severe Pediatric Cases in 2020. *Journal of Public Health Management and Practice*, 2020; 26(4):325-333. doi:10.1097/PHH.0000000000001190.

181.　　　Zahra Belhadjer, Mathilde Méot, Fanny Bajolle, Diala Khraiche, Antoine Legendre, Samya Abakka, et al. Acute Heart Failure in Multisystem Inflammatory Syndrome in Children. *Circulation*, 2020; doi:10.1161/CIRCULATIONAHA.120.048360.

182.　　　Ankit B. Patel, Ashish Verma. Nasal ACE2 Levels and COVID-19 in Children. *JAMA*, 2020; 323(23):2386-2387. doi:10.1001/jama.2020.8946.

183.　　　Leora R. Feldstein, Erica B. Rose, Steven M. Horwitz, Jennifer P. Collins, Margaret M. Newhams, Mary Beth F. Son, et al. Multisystem Inflammatory Syndrome in U.S. Children and Adolescents. *New England Journal of Medicine*, 2020. doi:10.1056/NEJMoa2021680.

184.　　　C. Galván Casas, A. Català, G. Carretero Hernández, P. Rodríguez-Jiménez, D. Fernández-Nieto, A. Rodríguez-Villa Lario, I. Navarro Fernández, et al. Classification of the Cutaneous Manifestations of COVID-19: A Rapid Prospective Nationwide Consensus Study in Spain with 375 Cases. *British Journal of Dermatology*, 2020. doi:10.1111/bjd.19163.

185.　　　Uwe Wollina, Ayşe Serap Karadağ, Christopher Rowland-Payne, Anca Chiriac, Torello Lotti. Cutaneous Signs in COVID-19 Patients: A Review. *Dermatologic Therapy*, 2020; doi: 10.1111/dth.13549.

186.   CDC COVID-19: Older Adults. Revised June 25, 2020. Accessed July 1, 2020. https://www.cdc.gov/coronavirus/2019-ncov/need-extra-precautions/older-adults.html

187.   Rachel M. Werner, Allison K. Hoffman, Norma B. Coe. Long-Term Care Policy After COVID-19—Solving the Nursing Home Crisis. *New England Journal of Medicine*, 2020; doi:10.1056/NEJMp2014811.

188.   CDC COVID-19: People of Any Age with Underlying Medical Conditions. Revised June 25, 2020. Accessed June 28, 2020. https://www.cdc.gov/coronavirus/2019-ncov/need-extra-precautions/people-with-medical-conditions.html.

189.   Smriti Mallapaty. Mounting Clues Suggest the Coronavirus Might Trigger Diabetes: Evidence from Tissue Studies and Some People with COVID-19 Shows that the Virus Damages Insulin-Producing Cells. *Nature*, 2020; 583:16-17. doi:10.1038/d41586-020-01891-8.

190.   Dominique J. Pepper. Obesity Survival Paradox in the Critically Ill. *Critical Care Medicine*, 2017; 45(8):e872. doi:10.1097/CCM.0000000000002474.

191.   Naveed Sattar, Iain B. McInnes, T John J.V. McMurray. Obesity Is a Risk Factor for Severe COVID-19 Infection: Multiple Potential Mechanisms. *Circulation*, 2020; 142:4-6. doi:10.1161/CIRCULATIONAHA.120.047659.

192.   Lynsey Forsyth. COVID-19 Severity is Increased in Patients With Mild Obesity. American Association for the Advancement of Science. Published July 15, 2020. Accessed July 17, 2020. https://www.eurekalert.org/pub_releases/2020-07/esoe-csi071320.php.

193.   Thijs Feuth, Tarja Saaresranta, Antti Karlsson, Mika Valtonen, Ville Peltola, Esa Rintala, Jarmo Oksi. Is Sleep Apnea a Risk Factor for COVID-19? Findings From a Retrospective Cohort Study. *medR$_x$IV*, 2020; doi:10.1101/2020.05.14.20098319.

194.   R. Pranata, A.Y. Soeroto, I. Huang, M.A. Lim, P. Santoso, H. Permana, A.A. Lukito. Effect of Chronic Obstructive Pulmonary Disease and Smoking on the Outcome of COVID-19. *The International Union Against Tuberculosis and Lung Disease*, 2020; doi:10.5588/ijtld.20.0.

195.   Marko Marhl, Vladimir Grubelnik, Marša Magdič, Rene Markovičb. Diabetes and Metabolic Syndrome as Risk Factors for COVID-19. *Diabetes and Metabolic Syndrome: Clinical Research and Reviews*, 2020; 14(4): 671–677. doi: 10.1016/j.dsx.2020.05.013.

196.   Zahra Raisi-Estabragh, Celeste McCracken, Mae S Bethell, Jackie Cooper, Cyrus Cooper, Mark J Caulfield, et al. Greater Risk of Severe COVID-19 in Black, Asian and Minority Ethnic Populations is Not Explained by Cardiometabolic, Socioeconomic or Behavioral Factors, or by 25(OH)-Vitamin D Status: Study of 1326 Cases from the UK Biobank. *Journal of Public Health*, 2020; doi:10.1093/pubmed/fdaa095.

CHAPTER XIII

197.   Frank L. Goldstein, Benjamin F. Findley Jr. Psychological Operations: Principles and Case Reports. Air University, Press Maxwell Air Force Base, Alabama. September 1996.

198.   George E. Vaillant. Involuntary Coping Mechanisms: A Psychodynamic Perspective. *Dialogues in Clinical Neuroscience*, 2011; 13(3):366-370.

199.   A. H. Maslow. A Theory of Human Motivation. *Psychological Review*, 1943; 50:370-396.

200.   Á. Zsila, R. Urbán, L.E. McCutcheon, Z. Demetrovics. A New Avenue to Reach Out for the Stars: The Association of Celebrity Worship with Problematic and Nonproblematic Social Media Use. *Psychology of Popular Media*, 2020; doi:10.1037/ppm0000275.

201.   Samantha K Brooks, Rebecca K Webster, Louise E Smith, Lisa Woodland, Simon Wessely, Neil Greenberg, et al. The Psychological Impact of Quarantine and How to Reduce It: Rapid Review of the Evidence. *The Lancet*, 2020; 395(10227):912-920. doi:10.1016/S0140-6736(20)30460-8.

202.   Wolfram Kawohl, Carlos Nordt. COVID-19, Unemployment, and Suicide. *The Lancet: Psychiatry*, 2020; 7(5):389-390. doi:10.1016/S2215-0366(20)30141-3.

203.   The plight of essential workers during the COVID-19 pandemic. *The Lancet*, 2020; 395(10237):1587. doi: 10.1016/S0140-6736(20)31200-9.

204.   Miia Jansson, Jordi Rello. Mental Health in Healthcare Workers and the Covid-19 Pandemic Era: Novel Challenge for Critical Care. *Journal of Intensive and Critical Care*, 2020; 6(2). doi:10.36648/2471-8505.6.2.6.

205.   Tawfiq Choudhury, Maciej Debski, Andrew Wiper, Amr Abdelrahman, Susan Wild, Shajil Chalil, et al. COVID-19 Pandemic: Looking After the Mental Health of Our Healthcare Workers. *Journal of Occupational and Environmental Medicine*, 2020; 62(7): e373-e376. doi: 10.1097/JOM.0000000000001907.

206.   Caitríona L Cox. 'Healthcare Heroes': Problems with Media Focus on Heroism from Healthcare Workers During the COVID-19 Pandemic. *Journal of Medical Ethics*, 2020; 46:510-513. doi:10.1136/medethics-2020-106398.

207.   Mohamad-Hani Temsah, Fahad Al-Sohime, Nurah Alamro, Ayman Al-Eyadhy, Khalid Al-Hasan, Amr Jamal, et al. The Psychological Impact of COVID-19 Pandemic on Health Care Workers in a MERS-CoV Endemic Country. *Journal of Infection and Public Health*, 2020; 13(6):877-882. doi:10.1016/j.jiph.2020.05.021.

Acknowledgements

Covid-19 Brain Team

Drs. Jawad F. Kirmani MD, Haralabos Zacharatos DO, Thomas Steineke MD PhD, Ashish Kulhari MD, Siddhart Mehta MD, Asha Iyer MD PhD & Amrinder Singh MD.

Healthcare Heroes

Spozhmy Panezai MD, Sara Strauss DO, Laura Suhan NP, Brigitte Percival NP, Daniel Rosenblatt MD, Lisa Casale MD, Namrata Baxi MD, Suman Bharath MD, Yong-Bum (Peter) Song Pharm. D, Gina Pagliaro PA-C, Anna Whetstone PA-C, Kathryn Patterson RN, Kraig Kirby RN, Brandon Poellot RN, Cleopatra 'Pat' Lapitan RN, Nancy DePinto Vassallo RN, Jacqueline Cabrera RN, Tina Evans RN, Fernanda Araujo RN, Linda Magvas RN, Kelly Ahearn RN, Lauren Huey RN, Sheena Liverpool RN, Denise Clark Edgeworth RN, Catherine Alexander RN, Gilda Sarnillo RN, Ingrid King RN, Arminda Mamaclay RN, Renee Henney RN, Naomi Starkman RN, Mike Kelton RN, Cindy Kiernan RN, Briana Decarvalho RN, Mike Kowalski RT, Kimberly Jones RD, Respiratory Therapy, Patient Care Technicians, The Proning Team, The Intubation Team, The Rapid Response Team, The Code Blue Team, The Dialysis Team, The PICC Team, Olga from Environmental Services, Aimee, Crystal, Desiree, and Debby (Miss D) from Food Services.

Thank You

Mom, Military Nurses, Girls Scouts of Central New Jersey & Edison High Cheerleaders.

ABOUT THE AUTHOR

Dr. Farah Fourcand, MD is a board-certified neurologist who trained at Georgetown University Hospital and the National Institutes of Health. She is the first person to complete the NIH physician-scientist track during her neurology residency and is currently in the only combined stroke, neurocritical care, and neurointerventional surgery program in the country. She is the only woman on this track and recently completed her stroke fellowship. At the peak of the COVID-19 pandemic, Farah became part of a COVID-19 Brain Team that treated ICU patients during the first wave of COVID-19. She is the study director of a COVID-19 clinical trial, continues to work on research in neurovascular conditions, and serves as a sub-investigator in present day landmark stroke clinical trials. Farah's research has also focused on neuroplasticity, neurorehabilitation, mitochondria in aging, population genetics, epidemiology, medical anthropology, and complementary and alternative medicine. Farah is a Tylenol Future Care Scholar, Gold Humanism Honors Society Inductee, and recognized for her contributions to neuroethics in medical education.

Farah is a Miami-native and received scholarships to the University of Miami and FIU Herbert Wertheim College of Medicine. As a medical student, Farah received the American Academy of Neurology Prize for Excellence and Community Medicine Service Learning Award. She served as House of Delegates Committee Chairwoman, President of the American Medical Student Association, led global health and health policy action committees, and was part of the team that spearheaded Miami's first mobile health clinic in underserved communities. Farah engaged in policy development for evidence-based medicine, innovation, and access to healthcare as well as advocacy for diversity in medicine, opportunity for people with disabilities, physician awareness of the LGTBQ+ community, and empowerment for underprivileged youth. She continues to advocate for stroke and traumatic brain injury survivors.

Farah currently lives in Metuchen, New Jersey with her fiancé Ryan, blind Siamese cat Butters Stotch, his one-eyed brother Ace Ventura PD, and Oliver Sacks. She enjoys painting, art history, cheese, food and hot sauce challenges, cooking, dancing, and wanderlust. Since a modeling agent discovered her during her internship, Farah moonlights as a fashion model and has been featured in publications such as Washington Life Magazine and walked in DC, San Francisco, and New York Fashion Weeks.